Beyond
Self Resistance
Bodybuilding
Course

Beyond Self Resistance
Bodybuilding Course

By

Birch Tree Publishing
Published by Birch Tree Publishing

© 2013 Copyright Birch Tree Publishing
Brought to you by the
Publishers of Birch Tree Publishing
ISBN-13: 978-0-9880821-0-6

Tables of Contents

The Beyond Self Resistance Manual was designed to showcase my gains with Hybrid Methods that explain various muscle-stimulating techniques in great detail. It essentially kick-started the Beyond muscle-building stress methods—and the gains of muscle-sculpting weight-free-trainees all over the world.

Preface By Ryan Mclean

For the masses, when it comes down to self resistance training whether it works or not or how to perform those exercises efficiently can be confusing. They have no idea how the exercises are to be performed or which exercises work, much less how to progress in a systematic manner without wasted effort. This book is designed to remove much of the hit-and-miss training misconceptions in regards to self resistance exercises. Granted, some experimentation will be needed due to individual structures, muscle length, recovery factors and so on, but the trial and error, have been eliminated for you.

For within your hands the material contained within these pages are based on sound validated data. Marlon Birch has dedicated a large portion of his life towards experimenting and eventually discovering the principals of efficient muscle-sculpting and strength building principals of proper (bodybuilding Strengthening Resistance Exercises). This book is arranged in a proper structure in order to reveal to the trainee how to benefit from self resistance exercises and how to use them properly to increase strength and size gains.

The question of which is the best way to utilize these exercises for efficiency of effort, increasing strength, and that chiseled hard look has been a controversial battle for some time. This book is designed for the hardgainer with less-than-favorable genes. This system categorizes exercises and routines, so the trainee receives total growth producing stimuli and maximum and efficient muscle fiber recruitment.

These stress methods and hybrid techniques, were used early in Marlon Birch's career to change his mediocre build to a build that impressed his family and friends. Each program supersedes the last and you will see and feel a difference. As you the trainee will notice what Marlon is offering within these pages is a new perspective on self resistance training, based not on the consideration of his peers or the bodybuilding community and commercial supplement industry. But, from solid science and thinking applied to self resistance strength training exercises.

INTRODUCTION

I think everyone knows my story by now from the Beyond Self Resistance Mini Introductory Course. However, Like most teenagers growing up surrounded by He-Man, Superman and Hulk cartoons and various comics, I had visions of being heavily muscular that would impress my friends and family. I've also had dreams of competing in bodybuilding competitions, and after a few years of my development being somewhat of a respectable level I decided to jump into the ring. I had fun with my first (play) contest, it never deterred me though, and I kept plowing along. Never losing faith and kept that dream of achieving it all in my minds eye. While I did improve on my physique from my first contest, the real progress that I longed for did not materialize regardless what I did.

Years later with continued experimentations and pouring over tons of physiology and biomechanic textbooks, I came across a few methods and missing elements that was missing in my education. By applying my newfound methods and extended set training tactics I was floored! Not only did I realize I'd hit it big but everyone around me was asking: "(Hey), what the hell are you doing boy?" I showed some of my friends the methods, some laughed, some tried it and realized themselves that the combination works and works quite well." So, this book is my starting point and how I won my very first bodybuilding contest. By learning how to contract and grow those hard to reach endurance-fast-twitch-fibers.

I'm sure most trainees posses far better genetics than myself and will achieve far greater results with this course. This book will indeed clear up many self resistance pit falls and misconceptions. So, let's get into some efficient muscle producing training. Volume builds muscles, regardless of what the gurus say. Volume increases and unleashes new muscle-pumping growth for hardgainer type builds. It is my belief that this book is a system and can be learned by anyone who is willing to put in the time and effort. However, the trainee should spend enough time mastering the logic behind the training protocol to grasp my approach to high-intensity training.

It is my belief that this book is a system and can be learned by anyone who is willing to put in the time and effort. However, the trainee should spend enough time mastering the logic behind the training protocol to grasp my approach to high-intensity training. That will allow the trainee in time to answer his or her training problems when it comes to self resistance type exercises. What works and what doesn't. However, for now simply follow and learn. For everything is laid out for you.

My main goal is not to shape views and confuse the trainee to a point where they wonder if this is fact or fiction. Any trainee can see for themselves the newest quick fad diet or exercise training program. What many fail to realize is that these commercials and commercial publications prime reason is to sell their products and apparatus. What I have to offer the trainee within this book is a new perspective on building health, strength and chiseled muscles that one can use. Not based on commercial considerations, but derived from the trial, error and sound science to muscle-sculpting research and sound thinking.

This book is not based on developing false promises of 20-inch biceps. No real training program or person can honestly offer that. What I've got here is a system of serious thought and when applied, will enable the trainee to develop their muscles to the limits of their potential faster than any other system at present. My program is based on volume-oriented routines, at medium-to-high intensity for optimal muscle fiber stimulation without exhausting the trainee's nervous system, causing over-training.

Training to positive failure is one of the keys to muscle growth stimulus, but for hardgainers that are high strung, we need medium to high intensity phases for long periods within the set to trigger a new growth response.
Be Prepared to Work it.

--Marlon Birch--

BEYOND SELF RESISTANCE

STRESS METHODS

WORKOUT PLAN

Featuring the Double Impact & Various Hybrid
Muscle-Building Methods

by Marlon Birch

CHAPTER 1

What is Self Resistance..
Tension and Force Output..
Muscle Building Observations

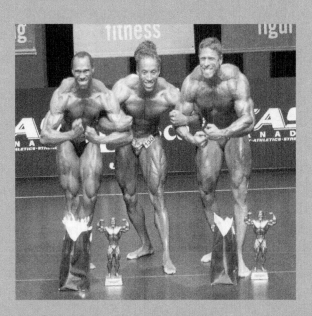

Marlon Birch Against the Mass Monsters IDFA 2008 2nd Place

CHAPTER 1

What is Self Resistance:

It's a unique type of training where one would use one limb to resist against another. A classic example would be to place your left hand onto the right wrist. Then pull up with your right as you resist with the left arm working your right bicep. When you reach the top of the movement, you push down with the left hand while resisting with the right working the left tricep. This form of exercise works the opposing muscle. On one arm you work the bicep and on the other arm the tricep.

Tension and Force

A trainee can increase their strength levels threefold by increasing the intensity of a muscle contraction. Once maximum contraction takes place training to failure isn't necessary. Now I'm not saying use brutal force here. That leads to connective tissue damage over time. This mini course allows the trainee to drive in multiple continuous tension gears that increases the contraction and force of every rep. Constant Tension increases muscle force and chiseled muscle growth. On a scale of 1-10 Ten being the hardest. 5-8 is best! That's an efficient form of training. Fast, Precise, Muscle Sculpting Tactics.

The Ideal Rep Speed for Chiseled Growth

The best rep speed for chiseled muscle development and strength is a two-three second positive and a two-three-second negative—In short up and down phase. Using a power cadence, which is one second up and one second down. Produce some serious strength gains within the musculature being trained. This faster rep speed suggestion (power cadence) causes extreme damage to more muscle fibers than slower traditional rep speeds. So what is the key? It's the forceful reversed turnaround for the one-to-two-second positive and negative movement.

That explosive jolt right at the semi-stretch stage of the targeted muscle activates significantly more muscle fibers, which force the muscle to continue firing, activating the stretch reflex and getting more dormant fibers into firing.

Main Goal

My main goal is not to shape views and confuse the trainee to a point where they wonder if this is fact or fiction. Any trainee can see for themselves the newest quick fad diet or exercise training program. What many fail to realize is that these commercials and commercial publications prime reason is to sell their products and apparatus. What I have to offer the trainee within this book is a new perspective on building health, strength and chiseled muscles that one can use.

Not based on commercial considerations, but derived from the trial, error and sound science to muscle-sculpting research and sound thinking. This book is not based on developing false promises of 20-inch biceps. No real training program or person can honestly offer that. What I've got here is a system of serious thought and when applied, will enable the trainee to develop their muscles to the limits of their potential faster than any other system at present.

My program is based on volume-oriented routines, at medium-to-high intensity for optimal muscle fiber stimulation without exhausting the trainee's nervous system, causing over-training. Training to positive failure is one of the keys to muscle growth stimulus, but for hardgainers that are high strung, we need medium to high intensity phases for long periods within the set to trigger a new growth response.

Volume builds muscles, regardless of what the gurus say. Volume increases and unleashes new muscle-pumping growth for hardgainer type builds. It is my belief that this book is a system and can be learned by anyone who is willing to put in the time and effort. However, the trainee should spend enough time mastering the logic behind the training protocol to grasp my approach to high-intensity training. That will allow the trainee in time to answer his or her training problems when it comes to self resistance type exercises. What works and what doesn't. However, for now simply follow and learn. For everything is layed out for you.

Here are the reasons for higher-set-medium intensity training that can increase chiseled muscle and strength.

1) Greater full-blown pumps in the targeted muscles to increase capillary bedding, which in turn increases chiseled muscle size.

2) The trainee trains within a complete range of motion in the push/pull system in all muscle structures.

3) Cortisol production is down. Which means less muscle eating (catabolic-muscle wasting) which high-strung hardgainers produce a lot of.

4) The trainee activates as many fibers as possible with a wide range of exercises. Hardgainers have an abundance of low neuromuscular efficiency. Meaning, their nerve-to-muscle connections or pathways are way below average. So, the trainee needs more sets to trigger their muscle building efforts.

Once the trainee experiments with volume-oriented routines, but remember volume, even at a low intensity, will not trigger overtraining as high intensity can. Low intensity builds muscle size and strength, high intensity builds strength but damage tendons over time.

Now I'm not saying don't ever increase the tension on your exercises. Please do. But, do not increase the tension to such a degree to cause tendinitis (Applying Too Great a Tension). Volume with intense contractions due to stress methods will stress the muscles enough to promote rock hard chiseled muscle development and strength.

This is the first of the series of my muscle-building protocol based on full-range muscle stimulation, with the get-bigger trigger of efficient force producing muscle-sculpting protocol.

• **Basic Exercises** - Muscle team work with the muscle-teamwork exercises. To trigger intense contractions.

• **Stretch Exercises** - Which has a significant force component for stretch over-load linked to fiber splitting to increase muscle growth.

• **Continuous Tension/Occlusion** - or blood-flow blockage, which has been shown to significantly increase size and strength via endurance-component expansion, like capillary beds.

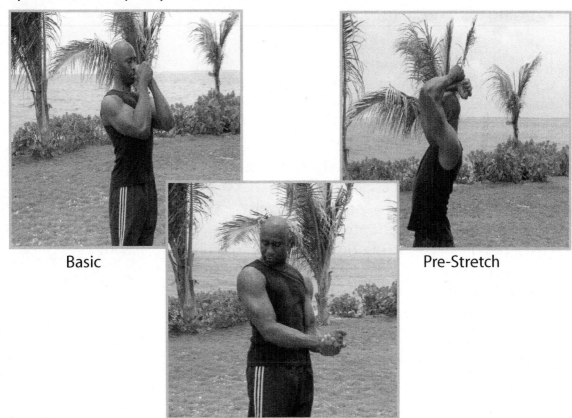

Basic   Pre-Stretch

Contracted

All of these critical components are necessary for developing any muscle quickly and completely. Multi-joint Basic Exercises are important as they hit the majority of muscle fibers in one go. The following explanation within these pages will be of benefit to the trainee. I've been a full range of motion trainee for many years with more than 25 years of exercise experience. The Beyond Self Resistance Series is simply using specific exercises that train each muscle through a complete range of motion. Igniting complete development within the muscle cells.

A great example would be the upper back. The basic and stretch exercise would be Three Chair Dips; it's a stretch-position exercise with a basic muscle component. Contracted-position movement would be Stiff-Arm-Pulldowns.

Here's the full muscle structuring overview:

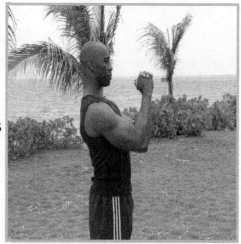

Basic: This is Muscle Teamwork, and it's the reason the big multi-joint exercises like decline pushups and three chair dips are so effective at packing on serious sculpted muscle. A number of muscle structures work together so you can drive up the entire musculature. This innervates the bulk of the target muscle, and they work as a team—they combine to generate the most force possible. Combined with self resistance strength-building exercises. The human body is designed to function as one unit. Which means that multi-joint, or basic, exercises are the best mass-building movements to increase growth and Fiber Recruitment.

Stretch: By incorporating an exercise that puts the target body-part in an overextended, or pre-stretched, state, like decline pushups for chest or three chair dips for the upper back, you can better activate the stretch-reflex. When the muscle is stretched, the nervous system sends an emergency response signal to the brain and a maximum number of muscle fibers are recruited. Using this pre-stretch reflex can help you get to fibers you couldn't recruit with other exercises. As well as causing the muscle to fire efficiently for the following exercises. Making your training session more productive.

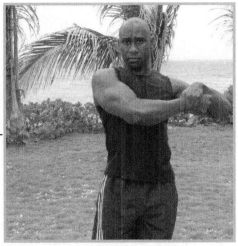

Across the Body Row

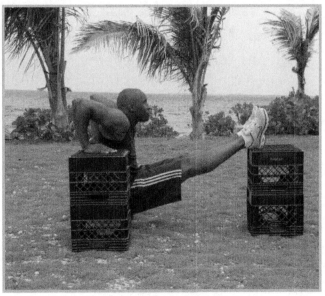

Three Chair Dips

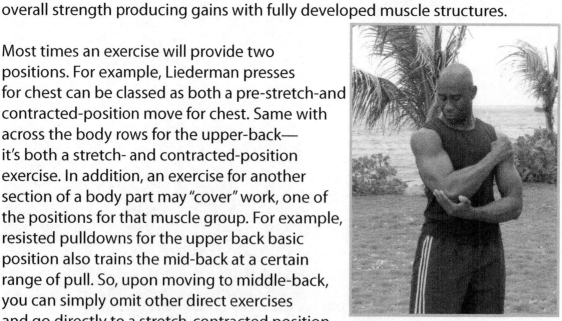

Contracted Exercises: Now that you have the majority of the fibers activated, you use an exercise that puts the target body-part in a position to contract against resistance which, produces tension and occlusion, or blood-blockage, a serious size-building routine with a tremendous cramping pump with no relief during the set (occlusion).

Once the set is finished, the muscle is engorged with a tremendous skin-stretching pump. For example, after forward extensions, you end your tricep routine with reverse-arm press-downs continuous muscle tension throughout the stroke. By training the three muscle producing positions —you work the target muscle through its full range of motion, which are key angles that coax overall strength producing gains with fully developed muscle structures.

Most times an exercise will provide two positions. For example, Liederman presses for chest can be classed as both a pre-stretch-and contracted-position move for chest. Same with across the body rows for the upper-back— it's both a stretch- and contracted-position exercise. In addition, an exercise for another section of a body part may "cover" work, one of the positions for that muscle group. For example, resisted pulldowns for the upper back basic position also trains the mid-back at a certain range of pull. So, upon moving to middle-back, you can simply omit other direct exercises and go directly to a stretch-contracted position.

How Much Tension

Tension or Progressive Resistance is the name of the game here. One need to be careful, and not overdo the tension. In order to understand we need to start at the top. The key principle the SAID principal. (SAID stands for Specific Adaptation to Imposed Demands). In short a trainee need to train with a variety of methods for the greatest amount of stimuli.

Getting a muscle to generate the strongest muscle building signal can be very difficult! With progressive resistance training maximum force is not necessary. It just needs to be strong enough. Also, Maximum tension isn't necessary to produce results with this form of exercise and is not advisable! As before, Resistance should be between 50-70 percent to increase muscle growth. Using a scale of 1 to 10. Ten being the hardest. Resistance should fall between 5-8. Most trainees would benefit from continuous reps of 15-20 within a 6-8 set count. In most cases with this amount of tension and reps, the muscle will appear to have increases in size and vascularity.

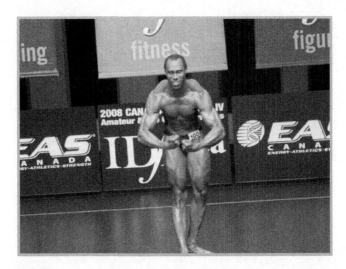

Marlon continues to progress with advanced Hybrid Stress Methods

CHAPTER 2

Bodypart Analysis

Neck Chest Upper-Back Mid-Back
Shoulders Biceps Triceps Forearms
Thighs Hamstrings Abs Calves

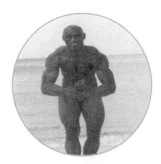

Neck

NECK AND UPPER TRAPEZIUS EXERCISES

The neck muscles and upper trap muscles are the most important muscles in the body apart from the lower back. The neck is very important and supports the weight of your head that's 8-10 pounds. All the neck exercises increases the strength, size and shape to the neck. As we say in the fitness world, alinement starts at the top! A well rounded neck/upper traps routine will enhance one's posture and maintain balance for the head.

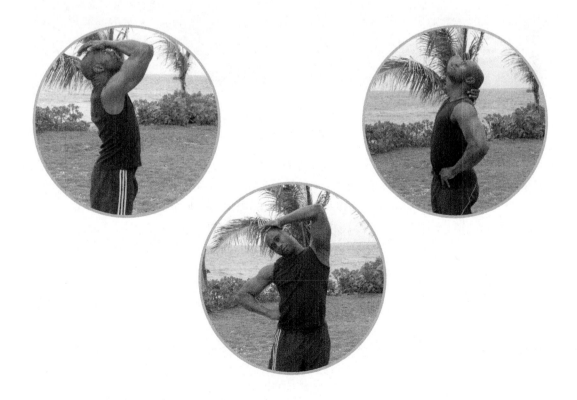

NECK AND UPPER TRAPEZIUS EXERCISES

Front Neck Press (Stretch and Contracted)

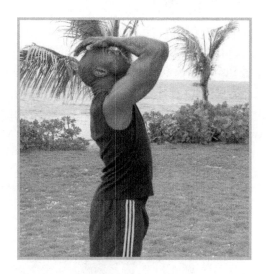
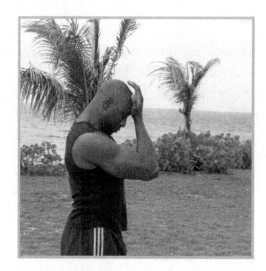

Start Position   Finish Position

With your head tilted back place your hand on your forehead. Now slowly press your head forward and resist the movement slightly with light tension towards your upper chest. Always use a light tension to the neck. As your strength increases use a little more force but not too much tension. Breathe Normal.

Rear Neck Press (Contracted)

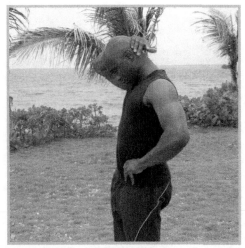

Start Position

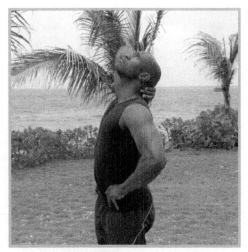

Finish Position

This movement is the opposite of the first movement. Place one hand behind your head and tuck the chin on the upper chest as shown. Now press the head against the hand while resisting with the hand until you're looking straight up. Use a light tension at the beginning and increase the tension to medium as you get stronger and more conditioned.

Side to Side Neck Upper-Trap Press (stretch)

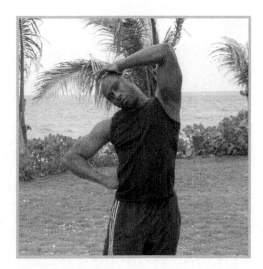 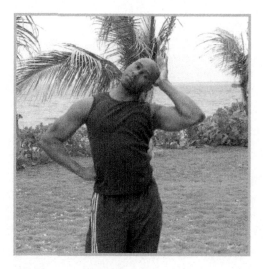

Start Position   **Finish Position**

Bend your head as close as you can to the shoulder as shown. Place the left hand on the left side of the head and press the head to the opposite shoulder while resisting with the hand. Followed by placing the right hand on the right side and press the head back to the starting position as before. Dual action left then right. Remember use a light tension and once the neck becomes more conditioned and stronger increase the tension.

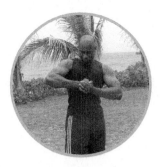

Chest

It's important to hit the chest muscles from many angles as possible to coax and force development. However, I learned that in order to really build a good chest it isn't one or two exercises it's a variety that will build the chest and increase it's strength! So in truth the best thing to do is to divide the chest in sections. Upper Chest, Inner Chest, Lower Chest. Instead of looking at it as a whole because it isn't. You must treat the upper and lower chest as two separate entities for your chest building venture to be a success. In my early years I did loads of pushups for the chest which hits mostly the lower and outer portions of the chest and do next to nothing for the upper chest. So I switched to decline pushups hands on blocks elbows in instead of out and the upper chest was taxed a great deal! So now my chest building starts with upper chest training. Giving priority to developing and stressing the upper chest.

Basic& Stretch: Decline pushups elbows in hands on a block works the upper chest really well. Along with help from the front portions of the shoulders and the tricep muscles.

Stretch& Contracted: Liederman Presses and Across the body presses really hit both elements in pre-stretching and increasing the peak contraction at the end of the movement. This position involves muscle-teamwork as well which will help the chest perform the movement. Help from the shoulders and triceps. Let's take a look at some muscle sculpting exercises.

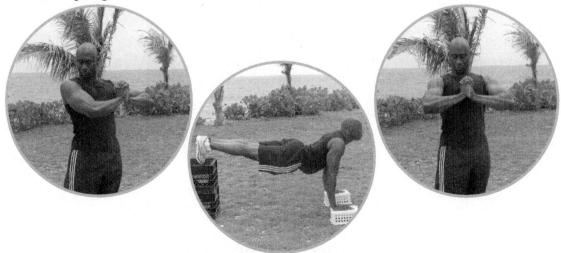

Upper Chest Press (Stretch and Contracted)

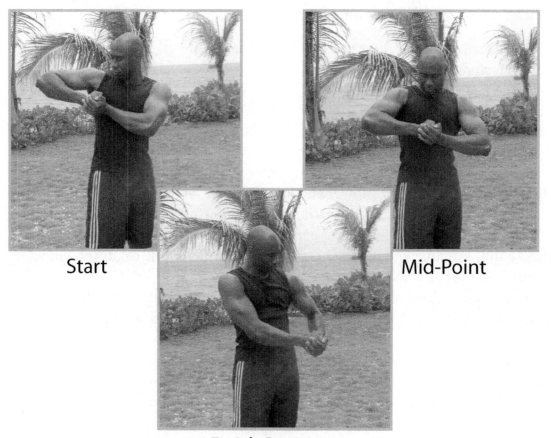

Start   Mid-Point

Finish Position

Place the right fist in the palm of the left hand as shown. Press the right hand down-wards resisting with the left hand until the right arm is across the body towards the left hip. Press the left hand upwards to the start position and repeat. Then change sides after all the reps are done. This exercise is a pre-stretch and contracted move.

Liederman Press (Stretch and Contracted)

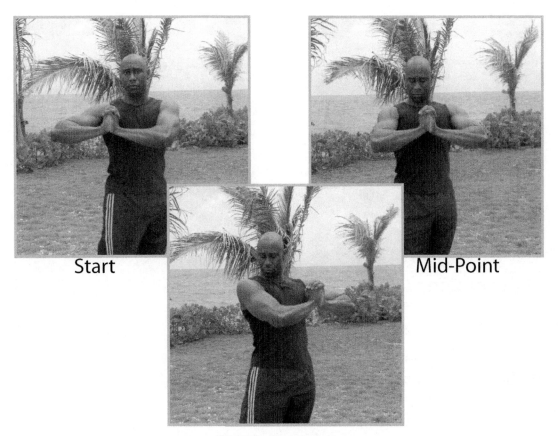

Start

Mid-Point

Finish Position

This is an Awesome building and shaping movement. Works the entire chest, lower, upper and middle chest as well as the shoulders and tricep musculature. Start off with the fingers interlocked as shown at the right armpit. Press right palm against the left palm towards the left armpit. Pause for 1-2 seconds and press the arm back and pause again before repeating.

Decline Push-Ups (Basic and Stretch)

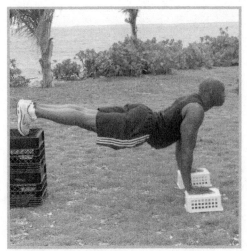 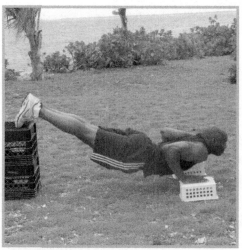

Start Position   Finish Position

This exercise is the Granddaddy of all upper-body exercises. An advanced version of the original Liederman pushup. This was his key upperbody exercise for the chest. It's the best upper-body builder and conditioner there is. This exercise is performed exactly as shown. Place your feet on a chair or box that's 10-15 inches high the higher you go the greater pre-stretch there is. At the bottom position to enhance muscle building stimuli pause at the bottom for 2-3 seconds before reversing the movement. Excellent for the upper and lower chest.

Three-Chair Pushups (Basic and Stretch)

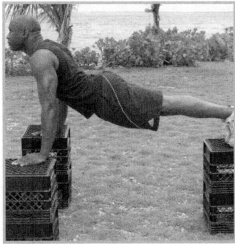
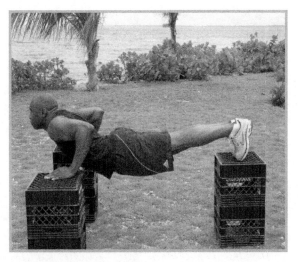

Start Position   Finish Position

This exercise is the Granddaddy of all upper-body exercises. An advanced version of the original Liederman pushup. This was his key upperbody exercise for the chest. It's the best upper-body builder and conditioner there is. This exercise is performed exactly as shown. Place your feet on a chair or box that's10-15 inches high the higher you go the greater pre-stretch there is. At the bottom position to enhance muscle building stimuli pause at the bottom for 2-3 seconds before reversing the movement. Excellent for the upper and lower chest.

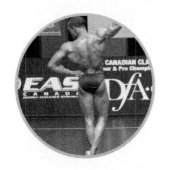

Upper Back/Mid-Traps/Lower Back

The structures of the upper back is quite powerful every point needs to be very carefully targeted. Basic Synergy Muscle Team Work, works well here. Thigh Rows, Resisted Pull-downs or Three Chair Dips are major corner-stone exercises to target the powerful upper back muscles. This will be explained within this chapter

Back Analysis

The upper back is very complex and house loads of different muscles com larger areas of the back the lats, upper neck and mid back muscles. This will hit the smaller muscles as well.The best way to start is to break things down into sections to see where what is targeting to really realize what you're doing and how to effectively target that large mass of muscle more efficiently.

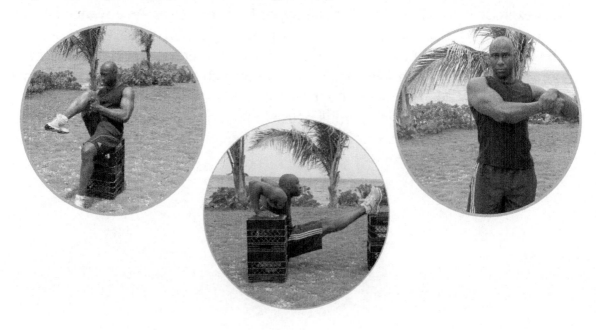

Upper/Lower Back Exercises (Basic)

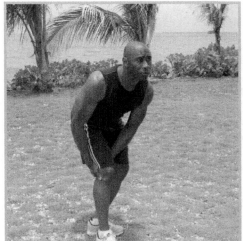

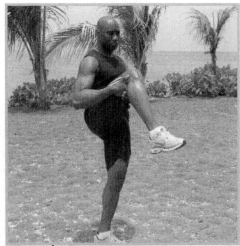

Start Position   Finish Position

Basic: Thigh Rows, these are perfect for targeting the upper and lower lat muscles as well as the lower back. Apart from that there's Resisted Pull-downs that targets the lats fully from top to bottom. These exercises are under continuous tension within the range of pull. However with the Thigh Rows resistance drops off a bit at the top position but by all means a highly effective exercise.

Interlock the fingers behind the knee as shown with right leg. With both arms pull the thigh upwards towards the chest while resisting with the leg.
This exercise widens the upper back, works the mid-back and stimulates the biceps as well. Work one side fully then switch to the other side. If balance is an issue perform the exercise standing against a wall.

Three Chair Dips (Basic/Stretch/Contracted)

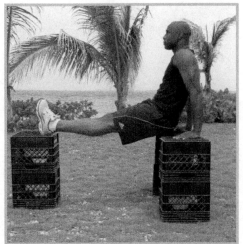

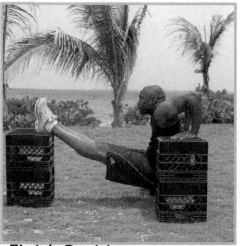

Start Position   Finish Position

As shown place each hand at least 15-16 inches apart, or shoulder width. Lower the body between the chairs pause one second and reverse the movement to the starting position. This is an awesome upper back widener.

Stiff Arm Pulldown (Contracted)

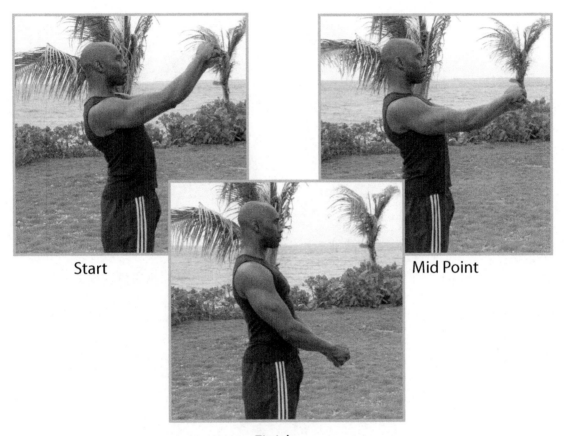

Start

Mid Point

Finish

Grasp the left hand with the right as in the picture. Gradually pull the arm downwards while resisting with the bottom arm. At finished position, Repeat by pressing the bottom arm up again by resisting against the top hand. Resisting in both directions for reps, then switch. Fantastic Upper and mid back strengthener.

Upper-Back/Mid-Back/Rear Delts (Pre-Stretch and Contracted)

Across The Body Rows

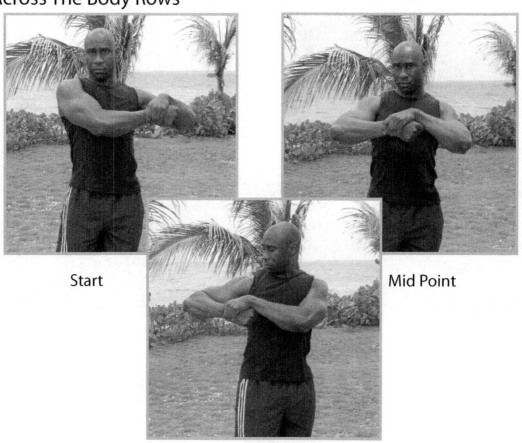

Start   Mid Point

Finish

Bring your right arm across the body pre-stretching the mid-back, grasp the wrist with the left hand. Slowly pull the arm across the body toward the right arm-pit against the resistance supplied by the left hand. Repeat the movement then switch arms. This adds thickens to the mid back and lats, along with the rear part of the shoulders.

Resisted Pulldowns (Basic and Contracted)

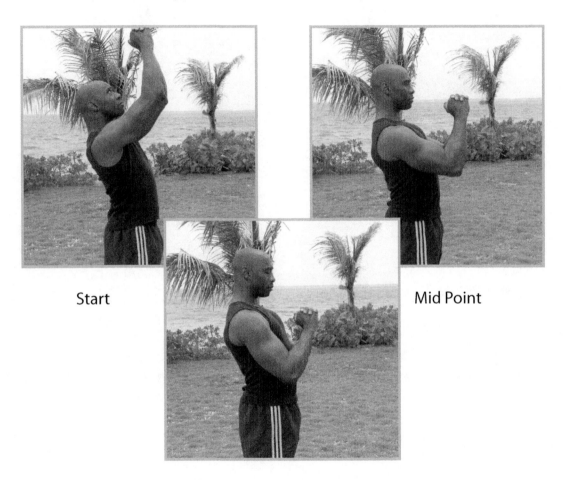

Start   Mid Point

Finish

With the arms overhead place your left hand on top of the right fist as shown.
Pull down with the left hand resisting with the right, once at finished position
press the right hand up resisting with the left hand for the desired reps.
Then switch arms. This works the entire upper back, biceps, and shoulders

Mid-Back Upper Traps (Contracted)

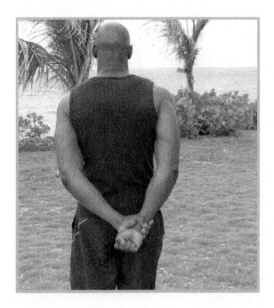

Start Position

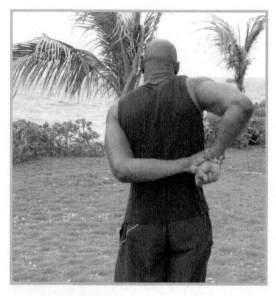

Finish Position

Place your right arm behind your back, hold onto the wrist with the left hand lean forward a-little and pull the right arm upwards while resisting with the left. When fatigue switch arms and continue. This works the mid-back,upper traps and rear delts.

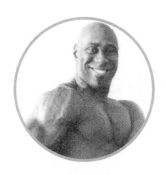

Shoulders

There's exercises that directly target the side head of the shoulders giving you that wide look. However at the very start I did an exercise that was just magic in terms of side and overall muscle development and strength. It's decline pushups hands on floor (elbows out). One can perform this by itself or with the isolation self resistance type exercises to add even more strength and muscle growth. Now it's been said that the lateral (side) will only be activated with lateral movements..but both forward and side resisted raises will stimulate the two heads.

The reason? One works with the other and they are intertwined with each other. The shoulder routine are packed with strength building and muscle pumping exercises that will create more width and roundness with efficient and muscle stimulating exercises. The shoulders contain three separate muscle heads, Front, Side and Rear heads. Lets take a closer look.

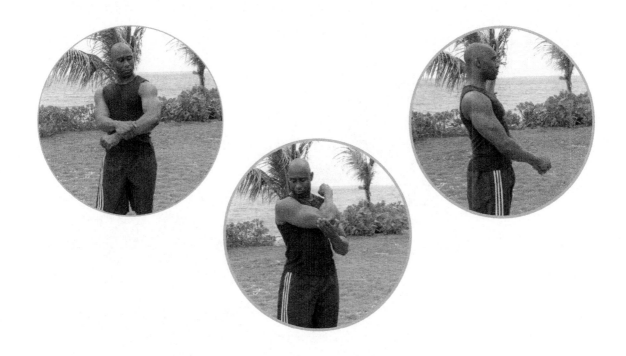

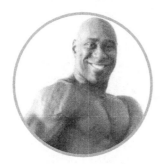

Shoulders

Shoulder Training & It's Effects

Now with all the pushing movements You'll be doing within this course you may think that you should lay off shoulder exercises a little seeing that almost all the upper body exercises contain some form of shoulder involvement. The shoulders, just like the calves and forearms. Constantly working.

Flexing and relaxing all day long when we walk, write/type, drive, lift a bag or put something on a shelf. Just like the upper back you need to separate the sum of parts and hit them in sections to really optimize your training when it comes to that area. Once separated precise and efficient training will surface.

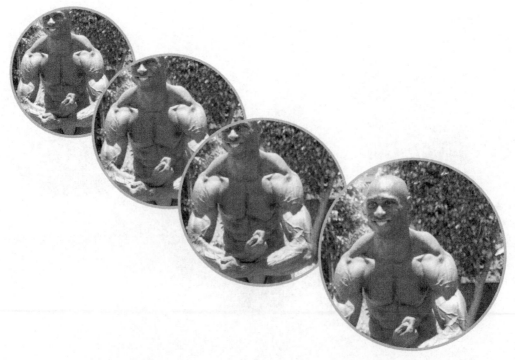

Decline Pushups (Basic)

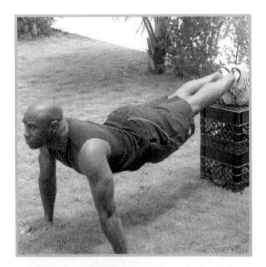

Start Position

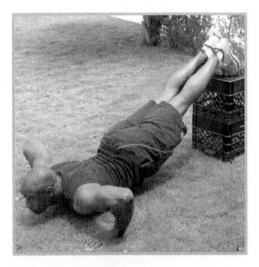

Finish Position

The Liederman Pushups.... This exercise is performed exactly as above. Hands on the floor, feet on a chair or stool at least 15 inches or more, the higher the stool the more the shoulders and upper chest work. Lower yourself as close to the ground as possible, then press back up again.

Across The Body Pulls Rear Delts (Contracted)

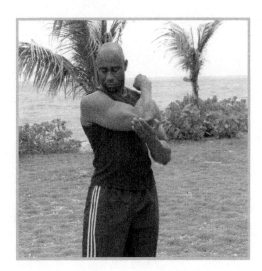

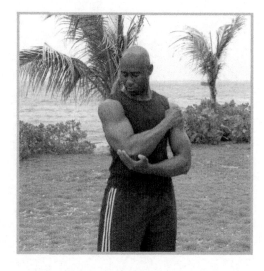

Start Position   Finish Position

Grasp the right elbow as picture shows firmly with the left hand. Slowly force the right elbow downward and backward while resisting with the left hand. Repeat for reps, then switch arms. This add great strength and development to the (rear) back part of the shoulders, lats and mid-back. It's best to start with this exercise first for it's easily neglected in a muscle-building program. As they say, Out of site out of mind.

Resisted Forward Raises (Contracted)

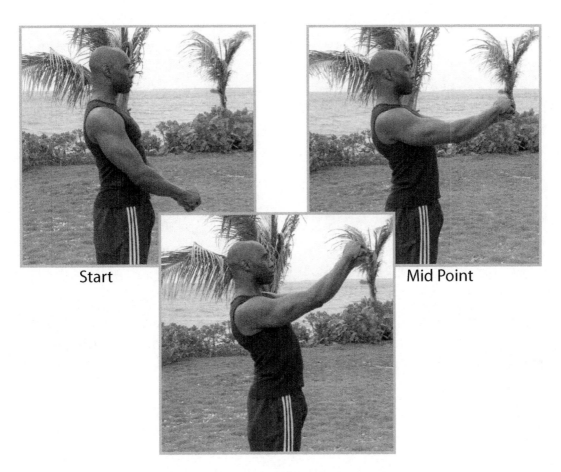

Start

Mid Point

Finish

Grasp the right hand with the left in front of the body as shown. Gradually raise the arm forward against the resistance of the other hand. Repeat for reps. Then switch arms and continue. This works the Front shoulder muscles.

Across the Body Lateral Raises (Stretch and Contracted)

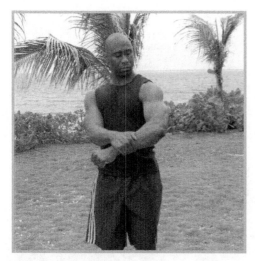

Start Position

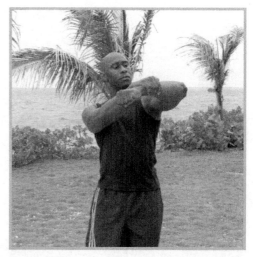

Finish Position

Grasp the left arm that is across the body as in the picture. Now raise the arm outwards towards the side contracted position resisting with the right arm. Perform desired reps then switch arms.

Resisted Shoulder Press (Basic and Contracted)

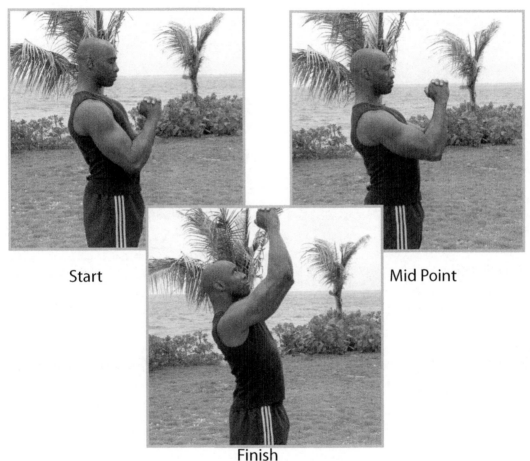

Start

Mid Point

Finish

Place the left hand on-top of the right fist. Press the right arm upwards while resisting with the left hand. Reverse the movement at the top by pulling the left hand downwards while resisting with the right. Continue for reps then switch arms.

Resisted Upright Pulls (Basic and Contracted)

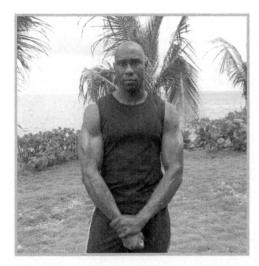

Start Position

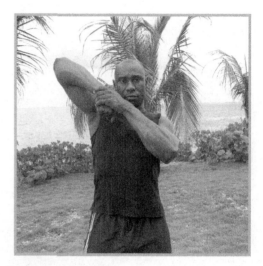

Finish Position

Hold onto the right wrist as shown above. Now pull the right arm upward while resisting with the left arm. Pull towards the ear, relax and repeat.

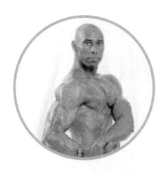

Bicep Training

Ok I've made a few changes to the original resisted curl to make it far more effective in building strength shape and muscle faster than before. At the very beginning while performing the original resisted curl gains were good but not great. Once I learned how to make the exercise harder and more efficient that's when my biceps and forearms really started to grow and take shape. It's all about efficiency in effort by changing this around to make it work better for you.

POWERFUL BALANCED ARMS

People are always looking at anyone that walk up that look a little fit or muscular, and what's the first thing they look at? The biceps and forearms. That's the first thing they see really. I've noticed it and all the people I've talked to about it have said so as well. It also helps when there's veins all around. What I've realized is that while I was developing or trying to develop my biceps and forearms my forearms got wider and was impressive when flexed , but my biceps looked narrow and when flexed flat looking. My biceps weren't as impressive hanging to my sides. It wasn't wide enough. So I paid attention to the exercises that would make a difference and one of the lessons I learned is to change the way I did the regular Atlas curls at different angles and hand positioning. This made a difference with increasing the diameter of my biceps.

Now when I stood, I looked at my biceps in the mirror it's the inner part of the bicep that gives that width! Height is another thing that the long head on the outside and the muscle that's under the bicep needs to be developed as well..the brachialis. Anyway, lets focus on what I did for the first phase then we'll break things down with the special Bicep and Tricep section later in this mini course. So here we go: Let's look at the muscle Sculpting exercises.

Bicep Curl (Palm Up) (Basic)

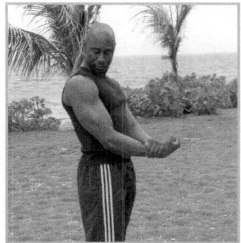

Start Position

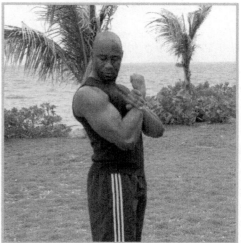

Finish Position

Grasp your right fist with the left hand. Pull the right arm upward towards the shoulder while resisting with the left hand. At the shoulder, reverse the exercise by pushing the left arm downwards resisting with the right. Continue for reps then switch arms.

Another Variation Palm Up Curls (Basic)

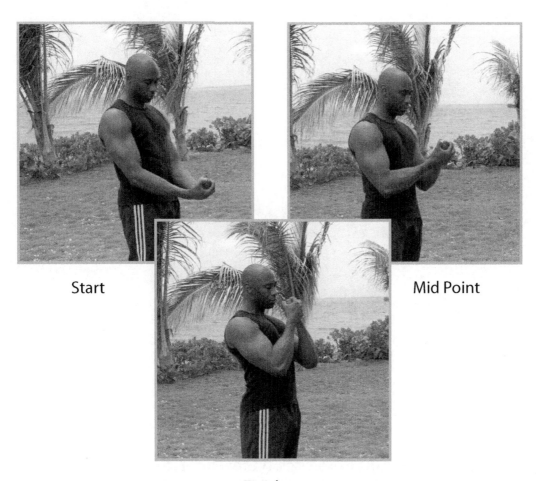

Start

Mid Point

Finish

This is another version of the palm up curl that's far efficient than the original version. This time place the left hand inside of the right hand. Now pull the right hand up towards the chest resisting with the left hand. Reverse the exercise at the top by pushing the left hand down resisting with the right for reps, then switch arms. This gives the biceps Awesome leverage for a greater bicep contraction.

Reverse Bicep/Forearm Curls

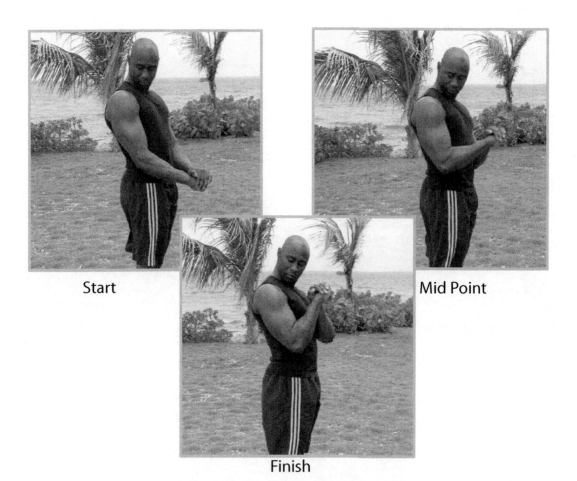

Start   Mid Point

Finish

This is the Grand-Daddy of all exercises. A Great bicep/forearm widener. Place the left hand on top of the right fist. Now pull the right arm upwards while resisting with the left hand. At the shoulder reverse the exercise by pushing the left arm downwards resisting with the right hand. Repeat for reps then switch arms.

Hammer Curls

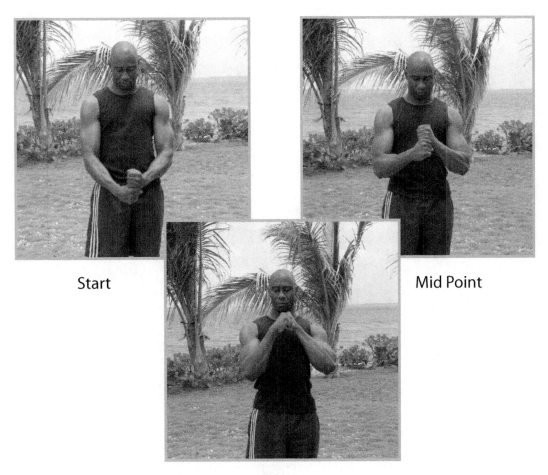

Start

Mid Point

Finish

Another great Bicep/Forearm combo. Place the wrists as shown in the picture above. Now pull with the right hand or bottom hand upwards to the chest while resisting with the top hand. At upper chest level reverse the exercise by pressing the top wrist down and resisting with the bottom wrist. Repeat for reps then switch arms.

Over-Head Curls (contracted)

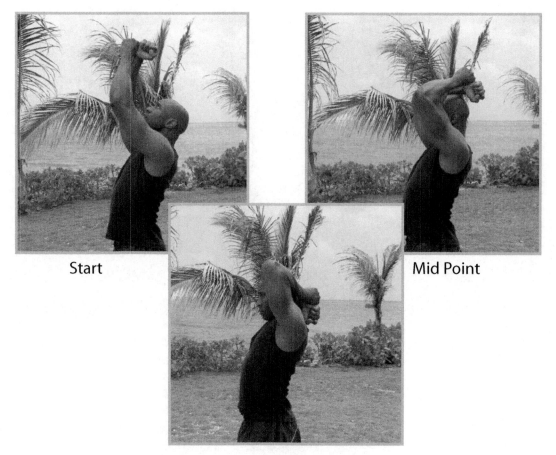

Start

Mid Point

Finish

This exercise stimulates the long head of the biceps increasing the bicep height and fullness. Place the hands in fists as shown. Now pull the top hand downwards while resisting with the bottom. Reverse the exercise by pressing the bottom hand upwards and resisting with the top. Use a moderate tension due to elbow sensitivity on this over head position.

Concentration Curls (contracted)

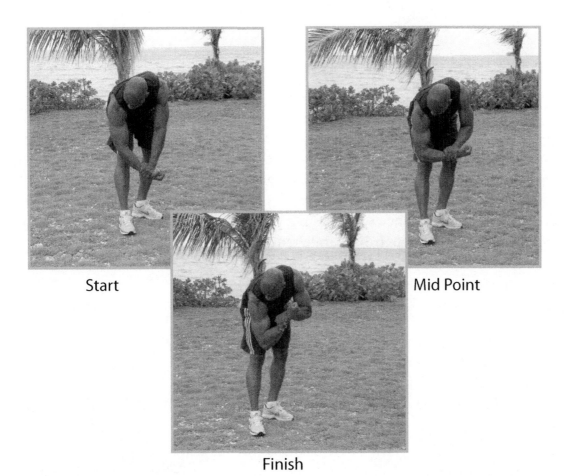

Start   Mid Point

Finish

This is a great bicep finisher move. Peak contraction to hit that long head again. As pictured in start position hold onto the right wrist with left hand and pull the right arm towards the face while resisting with the left hand. Now reverse the exercise by pushing the left arm down and resisting with the right.

Complete your reps then switch arms and repeat movement.

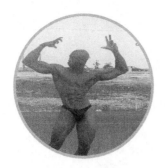

Triceps

The triceps long head is the largest part of the tricep musculature. It's responsible for the most tricep size. The tricep is broken into 3 muscle-heads. Lateral (outer head), Long Head (inside muscle), and the Middle or medial head. (middle muscle). The tricep is easily developed due to dips, pushups and a variety of self resistance type exercises. The self resistance exercises are geared to stimulate the tricep throughout the full range motion through 3 separate ranges of push.

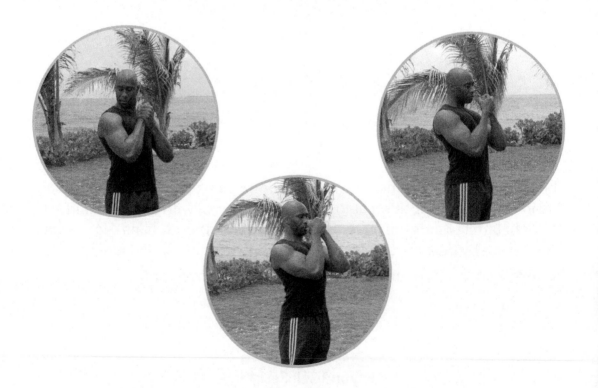

Forward Lateral Press (Basic)

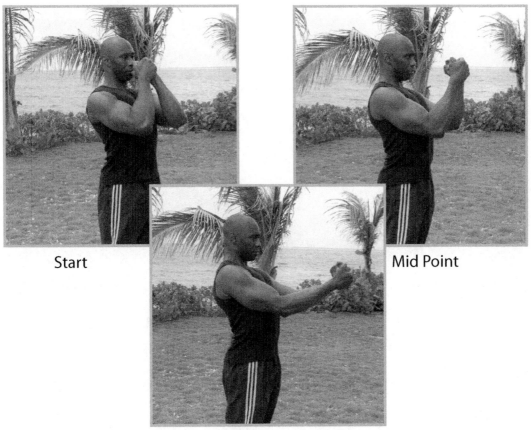

Start   Mid Point

Finish

Place the left fist in the right hand. Now push the left hand forward while resisting with the right hand. At the finished position reverse the movement by pulling the right hand towards you resisting with the left.

Tricep Pressdown (contracted)

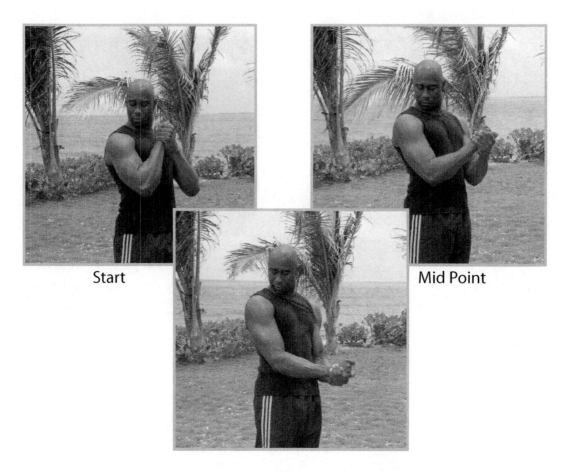

Start

Mid Point

Finish

Make a fist with the right hand and place it in the left. Now press the right hand downwards while resisting with the left hand. Repeat desired reps then switch arms.

Over Head Tricep Press (stretch, contracted)

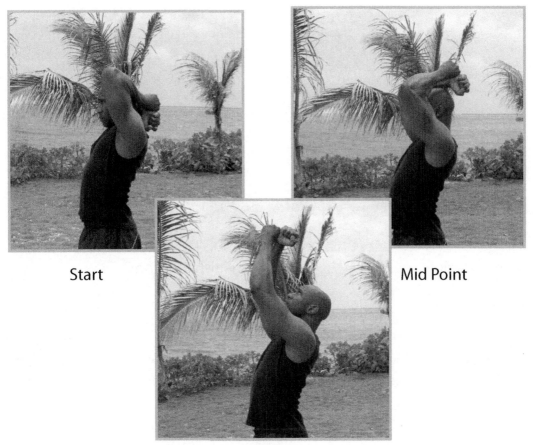

Start

Mid Point

Finish

Make a fist with both hands place it behind your neck. Now press the bottom fist upward while resisting with the top fist. At the top reverse the exercise by pushing downwards with the top fist while resisting with the bottom fist. Use a light to moderate tension due to the tricep tendons being quite sensitive at that position.

Decline Tricep Extensions (Basic)

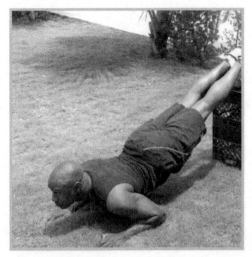 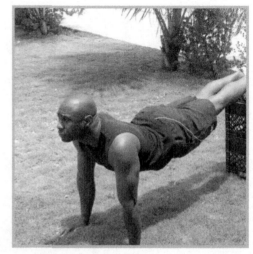

Start Position   Finish Position

Place your feet on a chair or box as shown in the picture. Place your hands and lower-arms on the floor and slowly press the arm straight out with a slight bend to the elbows. This exercise stimulates the outer head (lateral) muscle of the triceps.

Palm Up Tricep Press Down (contracted)

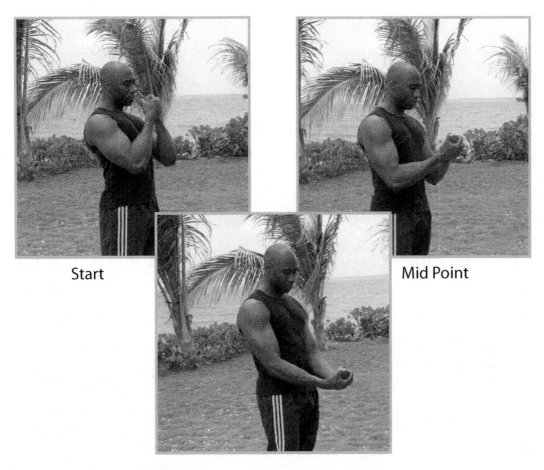

Start

Mid Point

Finish

Place the left fist palm up in the right hand. Now press the left hand downwards resisting with the right hand. Relax and repeat movement.

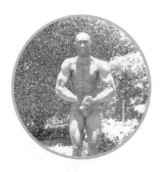

Forearms

Powerful forearms just like upper arms command respect! This muscle needs to be balanced with the upper arm. Last thing you want are forearms that look weak with powerful upper-arms. So, here's a number of exercises to increase the griping strength, and overall musculature of the lower arm, connective tissues of the wrists and increases and strengthens the grip.

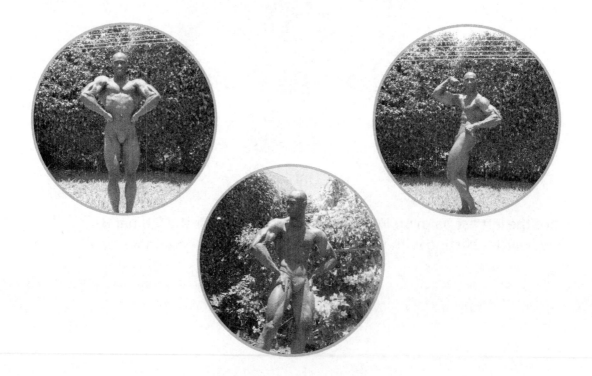

Palm Up Wrist Curls

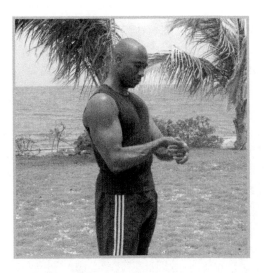

Start Position

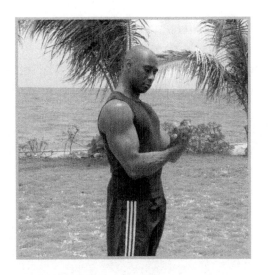

Finish Position

As pictured extend the right wrist backwards placing the left hand pressed against. Now Flex the right wrist upwards while resisting with the left hand. Practice till tired or desired reps are done then switch hands and repeat.

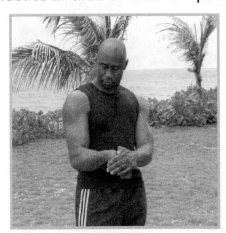

Start Position

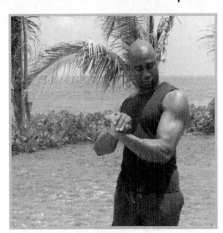

Finish Position

Same as before but this time the palm in pressed down. Resist with the opposite hand for reps then reverse hands.

Hammer Curls, Reverse Curls and Forearm Presses

The brachialis muscle that runs under the biceps and into the forearm, is the one muscle that's strongly targeted here. Resisted hammer curls and reverse curls gets the job done with a bicep effect as a tag-on! So these two exercises are the best efficient (basic) forearm-bicep exercises. These two exercises were covered earlier in our bicep exercises. So here we go again.

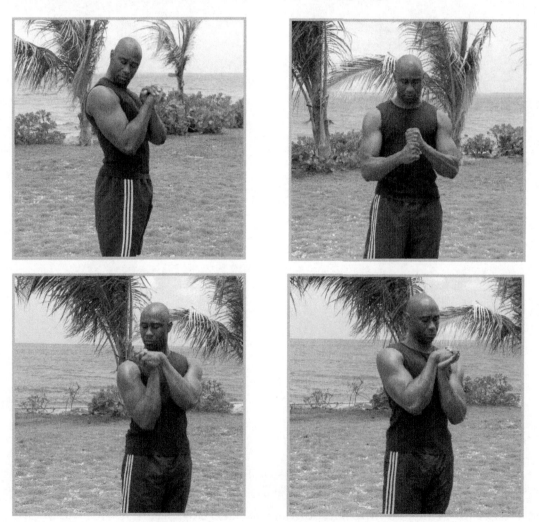

Perform this exercise as pictured by pressing to one side then the other while resisting with the opposite hand.

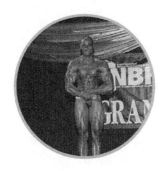

Thigh and Hamstring

Ok let's focus on the Powerful thighs and hamstring development exercises. Developing strength and power is what every athlete as well as every person wants. How do we achieve that? Let's start from the very top: One Legged Squats the King of All Lower-Body exercises stimulate everything! Thighs, Hips, Hamstrings, Inner Thighs and Glutes (butt). Followed by Leg extensions, and leg curls we are talking maximum efficiency. Multi-Joint exercises that stimulate the important hips, thighs and glutes is all we need. Let's get on with it..

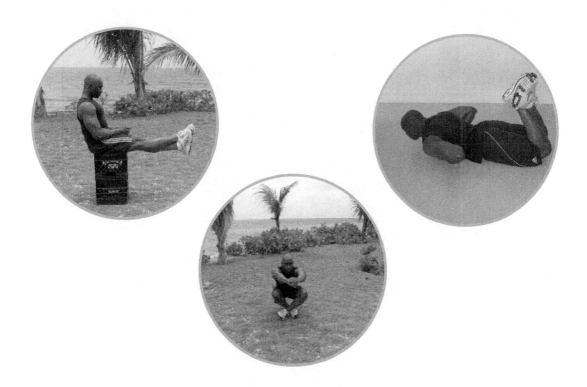

One Legged Squats

Few exercises are as impressive as a properly conducted one-leg-squat. Some of the best athletes and strength coaches in the world are unable to perfrom a single rep of this advanced exercise, let alone a full set of them. In time, though, with solid practice you will develop an awesome pair of muscular thighs, hmstrings and inner thighs to go along with it.

Stand with your knees slightly bent and your arms outstretched to balance. Lift one leg off the ground and place it as far out in front of you as possible while keeping it straight. (don't worry you will get better in time). Then, slowly lower yourself as far as possible on your balancing leg. When your hamstrings touch your calves (or as far as you can perform this exercise at first), push back up with the supporting leg to the start possition and repeat.
If your balance isn't tip top perform the exercise holding onto a chair with a free hand for support.

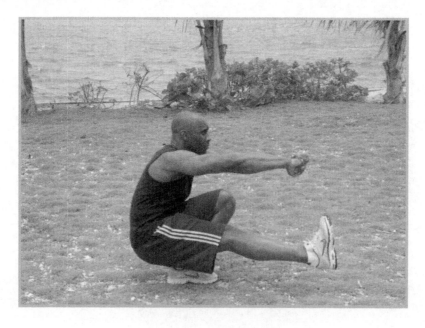

Crossed Feet Squats

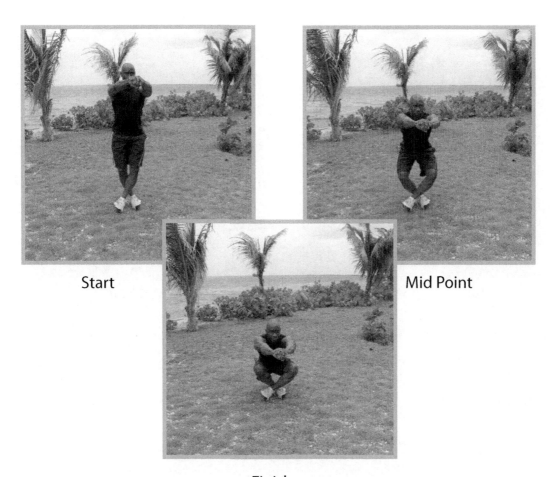

Start   Mid Point

Finish

Another excellent exercise for the overall thigh and hamstrings. Start off as shown in the starting position with feet crossed. Slowly under control lower yourself to the finished position No Bouncing one second pause then reverse the movement to the starting position. This exercise may be difficult at first but keep practicing and as night follows day it gets easier!

Resisted Leg Extensions

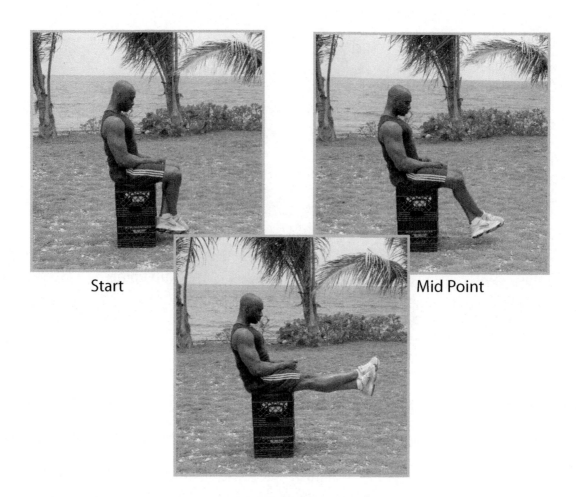

Start   Mid Point

Finish

While seated on a chair, box or stool, place the right leg over the left as shown in the picture, and extend the left leg outwards resisting with the right. At the top reverse the movement by pulling down the right while resisting with the left.

Hamstring Resisted Leg Curl

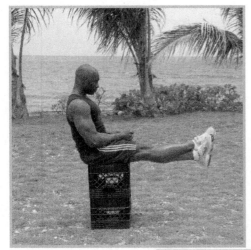

Start

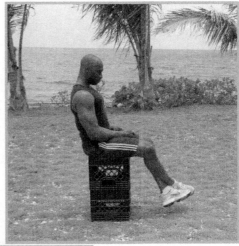

Mid Point

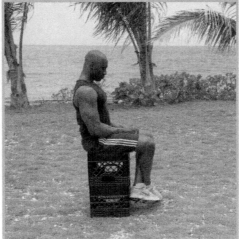

Finish

Just like the leg extension exercise, but the reverse. At the start position
pull the top leg down only resisting with the bottom leg. Repeat for reps.

Resisted Lying Leg Curls

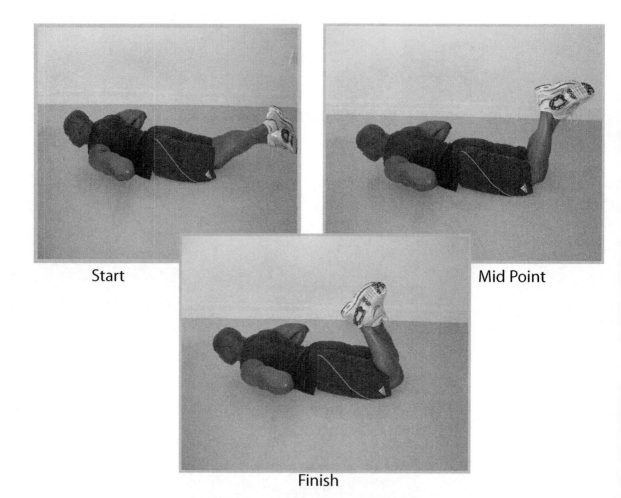

Start   Mid Point

Finish

While on the stomach on the floor place the left leg over the right as shown,
Now pull the right leg upwards towards you while resisting with the left leg.
Pull on the Up phase only. Repeat for reps then switch legs.

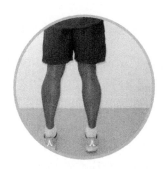

Calve Training

Now calf growth due to the dense layers of the muscles itself is quite stubborn! So my results within this department wasn't the best. However, I've learned a few things. In order for my calves to improve various steps had to be taken into consideration. I did loads of high reps daily but lost the true meaning of building muscle within this area. In order to add muscle onto those it's best to really focus on how you're doing the exercises and what rep range you're using for ultimate muscle building stimulation, which I'll explain in a moment). Here they are:

Stretch: You achieve this position at the bottom of any calf exercise—calves stretched off a high block. It's important to get that stretch to force the calves to contract at it's maximum!

HIGH REPS. As I've said earlier the calve is one dense muscle. The majority of these calf fibers are Endurance Oriented Fibers. Because it's used daily. You contract these muscles all day by walking. So they need to be taxed a certain way. The best way to target the calves are with reps that hit the range between 30 to 35 reps per set. Tension times are increased for your straight sets of calf work and should be about one minute or more, to efficiently hit the dense fibers effectively.

FEEL. As with any muscle group you must pay attention to the feel and focus on the muscle at hand. It is important to avoid bouncing and fast reps. Rep speed is also important. Three seconds up and the same speed for the down portion is about right. But feel is the most important element here. Another key to maximizing calf development and to increase the stress is to maintain the tension on the calve muscles.

By not coming all the way up to full contraction this maintains constant tension on the muscle and increases blood blockage. This will indeed increase growth stimulation, capillary development and muscle overload and what about the bottom range? This is just as important. It's important to get a max stretch at the bottom of the movement. This really pre-stretches the muscles to fire more efficiently due to the powerful stretch that loosens up the fibers, which produces additional growth.

More Calf-Growing Details

Now guys I don't have genetically superior calve development. Well not yet anyway..still working on it. After my experiment I added a component that was never done for my calves effectively, but last year my calves got even better than the year before with less work per set. They looked almost two inches bigger. It didn't make sense really. So I introduced a number of techniques and stress methods into my calve workouts for the first time

To see the effects of it all. Lo and behold my calves responded far better to the stress methods. After all, my calves looked much better with more size and shape and increased vascularity more naturally. Now I'm not blessed with inner-calf flare. So seeing that the methods increased that fact I loved it to the max!
By doubling up on the key contracted point of the movement with mini reps at the end of my full reps made the set far more intense. That's only one method I did. You will see more in later chapters in the routine sections.

Standing Calve Raises (stretch and contracted)

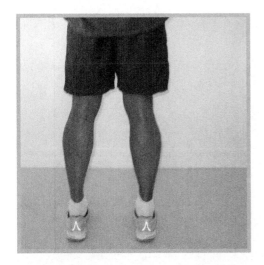 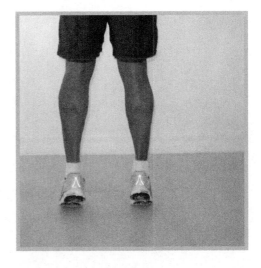

Start Position   Finish Position

This exercise can be done on the stairs or block. Start as shown and go up and down contracting the calves at the top of the movement. If on stairs, extend the heels as low as you can to really pre-stretch the calves, then press upwards into the contracted position. (finished position)

Slanted Pre-Stretch Calve Raises

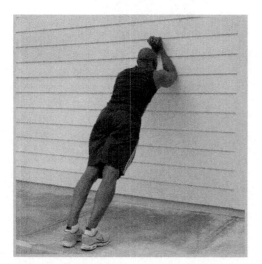

Start Position

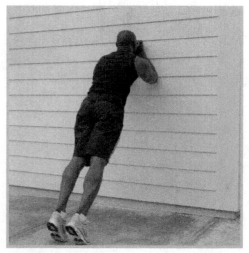

Finish Position

Stand at least 30 inches away from the wall, or position yourself as shown but make sure the calves are well stretched. Start off as shown in the picture start position. Press straight up on the toes then lower. This is as awesome calve stretch exercise. Perform this exercise until the calves are well tired.

This stimulates the entire calve.

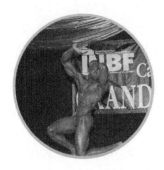

Abdominals

Abdominal Training are endurance type fiber muscles. Very much like forearms and calve muscles. Which means they need longer tension times and high rep ranges to benefit from training.

Muscle Makeup: The abdominal muscles are just that—muscles. It's one sheet of muscles with tendons dividing the muscles into blocks. So, it isn't upper and lower it's one sheet. Each is made up of the same types of fibers as your biceps, chest and back; however, as I mentioned, many of the fibers in the abs are more endurance oriented and require higher reps to reach full development.
The main abdominal muscle that one need to be concerned with, is the rectus abdominis, (front area) this isn't a bunch of knotted musles, as it appears to be, but rather a sheet-type muscle that runs from the bottom of your rib cage and attaches to your pelvis. As I've said earlier, The ripples are actually caused by tendons running horizontally and vertically. Throughout the entire length that cause the block type muscle separation you see.

Hip Flexor Function: The hip flexors come into play on many ab exercises, such as reverse crunches. As you'll soon see, the hip flexors are important contributors, when you exercise the rectus abdominis. Upper and lower separation. Like I said, there's no real separation on upper and lower abs. Studies indicate that the upper rectus abdominis can work somewhat independently of the lower part of the muscle, as it does when you perform crunches. Or abdominal situps
(feet extended not anchored) But when you work the lower portion, your upper rectus always comes into play, as in reverse crunches or across the body crunches.

Therefore, you should always work the lower area first, which brings both upper and lower sections into play. If you isolate the upper part first, you fatigue that area and make your lower-ab work much less effective—in much the same way that working forearms before biceps can limit your biceps efforts. For example, if you do crunches first and then reverse crunches, which works your upper rectus will be so fatigued from the crunches that it'll cause you to fail on the Reverse Crunches long before you fatigue your lower abs—it's one reason so many trainees lack lower-ab delineation:

They work lower abs last or do only crunches in their ab program. So here's just a few exercises that gets the job done. It works the muscles in union in order to get the best of both worlds.

Reverse Crunches

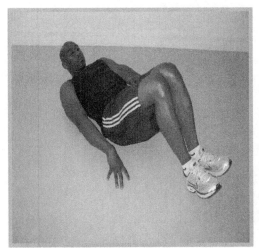

Start Position

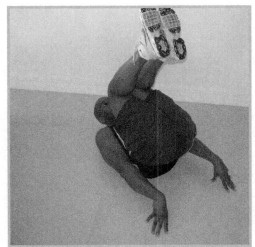

Finish Position

Start as shown in the start position picture. Then roll the hip as you bring the knees into the chest and continue for desired reps.

Across-The-Body Situps

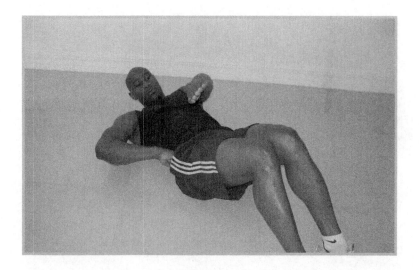

Start Position

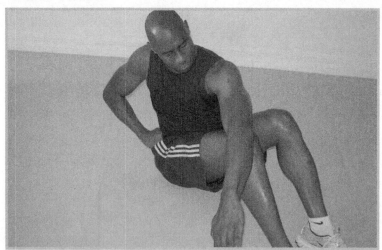

Finish Position

Start as shown in first picture. Now raise the upper body upwards and extend the left arm across the right knee as shown. This is a fine exercise for the entire abdominal wall as well as the obliques. After working one side for reps continue with the other in the same manner.

Beyond Self Resistance 72

Across-The-Body Side Crunches

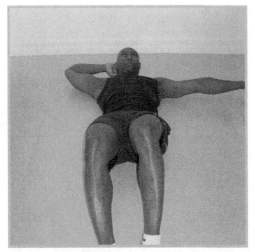

Start Position

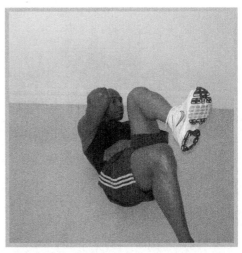

Finish Position

Start off flat on the floor with right hand by the ear or behind the head, Knees together feet on floor, place the non-working arm on the floor or on the stomach. Now, rotate towards the left knee as shown while bringing it towards the elbow. While touching reverse the movement by going down and lowering the foot in line with the other leg. Perform for reps then change sides.

Another Version

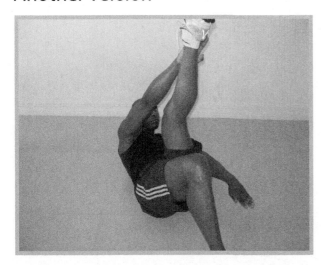

Stiff Legged Presses

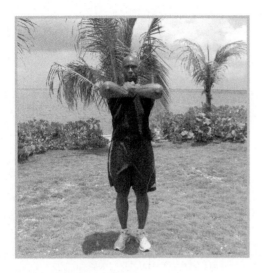

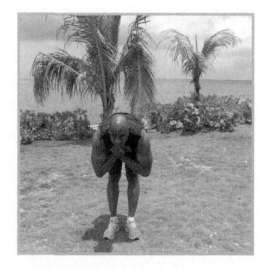

Start Position   Finish Position

Place the hands on your chest. Now, press downwards while resisting with the hands until you are in the finished position. Relax and repeat for reps. This pre-stretches the hamstrings and adds strength to the lower back musculature..

STRESS METHODS

Ten by Ten Method
Double Impact Method
Compound Isolation Method
Fiber Overload Method
Double Dip Stress Method
20, 20, 20 Stress Method

Stress Methods

Ten by Ten Method: Perform this stress method by performing ten complete full reps immediately followed by ten half reps from the start position to mid-point.

Double Impact Method: Perform this stress method by alternating one full rep immediately followed by a half rep. (one full and one half equals one rep)

Compound Isolation Method: Perform three sets of one exercise by itself. Then superset two other exercises. A superset is combining two movements back to back and then you rest.

Fiber Overload Training Method: Perform the exercise at the strongest muscle building signal, the Power Point. This means you are only training to the half point. Using the curl as an example, you curl from the starting position to the half way point, stop, and then push back down. Or with the push-up. You start at the bottom position you push half way up and then come back down again.

Double Dip Overload Stress Method: A perfect example to describe this method would be to perform a curl from the start to mid-point, lower the arm perform another half rep followed by a full rep. so, two half reps followed by a full rep.

20,20,20 Stress Method: This method increases fiber density overload. Perform 20 reps at the start to mid-point position, followed by another 20 reps full range, then finally a last 20 reps from the start position again to mid-point.

CHAPTER 3

Fiber Density
and

Neuromuscular Efficiency

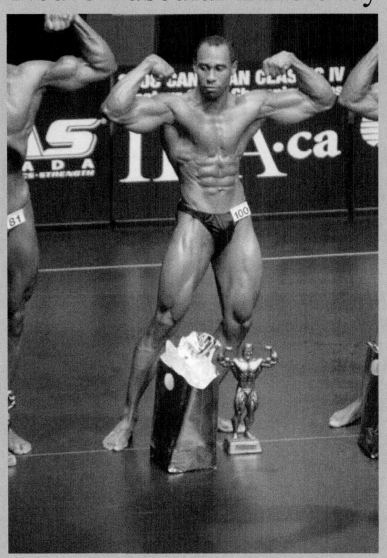

Neuromuscular Efficiency, which refers to the nerve-to-muscle connections, is important for contraction strength. Weak nerve-to-muscle connection is the sole reason hardgainers do not benefit from their contractions.

Now there is nothing one can do to alter fiber density of the muscle (meaning muscle thickness). However, the trainee can improve their neuromuscular efficiency by using a phase approach of volume-oriented sets and reps. Performing more sets and reps conditions the system to fire more muscle fibers within the contracted position.

Fiber density, like muscle length, determines the potential size of that muscle. Naturally thin (hardgainer) type trainees may contract 20 to 40 percent on an all out exercise. There's many ways on increasing the capacity to activate over 50 percent of fibers. It isn't increasing tension, it is learning how to increase the contractile capacity with an intense exertion per rep.

It is a fact that high tension resistance moves do little for muscle size increase, and will show little improvement in the trainee's muscularity and tendon health. Low to medium intensity work and learning how to contract the muscles efficiently, will not only stimulate more fibers to fire rapidly, but, will stimulate the trainee's ability to become more proficient to contract the muscles with more power output.

In short, with high intensity contractions the set ends too short and such tasks do very little to stimulate the endurance fibers to grow. Medium contractions are the most important requirement for stimulating muscle size and strength gains. Remember, the All or None Law in Beyond Self Resistance Mini Course? If the contraction is too great, the muscle fibers will not fire. Resulting in no muscle stimulation.

More-over, extreme high intensity contractions prevent the trainee from reaching those hard to get endurance fibers, thus producing no muscle growth and tendinitis. For once, a trainee tries high intensity work sets, they will realize it isn't possible to procure sure contractions within the extended growth threshold self resistance trainees need. Which ranges from 35-45 seconds on tension time.

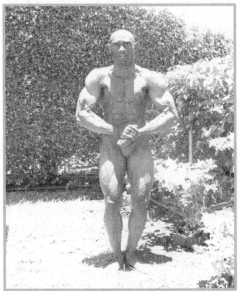
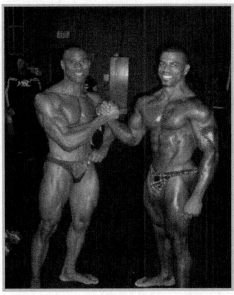

Pictures Above: Marlon kicks butt and continues to stress the natural and un-natural compeditors worldwide. They have no idea Marlon do not lift weights, and have followed the self resistance form of training and have developed various Hybrid methods that enhanced his physique.

Ten By Ten Force Production and Muscle Growth

Startling size and strength gains can happen when you merge time under load and tension at every workout because you train both components of the key high-growth endurance oriented muscle fibers. It's a serious size-building protocol—muscle force plus endurance-component expansion—that can take your muscle size to a new size and fullness within focused muscle-sculpting-training phases.

I've combined the emphasis on developing the myofibrils with time under tension muscle-force generating many actin/myosin strands in muscle fibers within the work set. This increases muscle density due to longer tension times, or doing more work in less time by performing the Ten by Ten method—more on that in later chapters). The Ten by Ten Method focuses on expanding the sarcoplasm, the energy fluid inside muscle fibers where glycogen, ATP and the mitochondria reside.

Both tension time and density are important if you're after maximum muscle stimulation and growth. Dual-capacity fibers with both a power/density and endurance component need to be trained that way. With extended sets and reps to promote enough muscle stimulation to increase size and strength within the muscles. Unfortunately however, most trainees have been brainwashed into thinking that they must use heavy resistance and lower-rep ranges for muscle growth and strength gains. That's one of the big reasons muscle gains are very slow for the majority of trainees, along with sore tendons and ligaments due to overuse. It's also the reason that I've developed the Ten By Ten Training method, along with other hybrid-stress-methods.

You the trainee will receive a massive pump and growth spurt. Why? Because most trainees neglect to stimulate the endurance fast twitch fibers at every workout. Now, what is the Ten By Ten Method? Here's a synopsis: let's use the bicep curl. You simply start the movement performing 10 powerful full reps, immediately followed by another 10 reps from the bottom of the curling movement to mid-point. Which is the strongest and most beneficial point within the curling motion. This increases excruciating pain and a full-blown pump within the muscle fibers.

When I tried this method of force production in my experiments in 1995, I realized the myofibrils got thicker with the combined tension-occlusion expansion within the working set. It's a serious extended combo to grow type training protocol. However, I will present the full program I used and the updated method of the Ten by Ten Method that I've refined throughout the years. It's one of the most effective size and strength builders there is. Simply because it increases force generation and extended tension times for those hard to stimulate endurance fast twitch power fibers.

That's specificity of training, or focusing on both aspects of the 2A power and endurance fibers within the workout. It isn't the 2Bs power fibers, as we have been led to believe throughout the years. It's the Fast-Twitch Endurance-Oriented 2As which have both muscle-building and endurance properties.

This is the first of the series of my muscle-building protocol based on full-range muscle stimulation, with the get-bigger trigger of efficient force producing muscle-sculpting protocol.

• **Basic Exercises** - Muscle team work with the muscle-teamwork exercises. To trigger intense contractions

• **Stretch Exercises** - Which has a significant force component for stretch overload linked to fiber splitting to increase muscle growth.

• **Continuous Tension/Occlusion** - or blood-flow blockage, which has been shown to significantly increase size and strength via endurance-component expansion, like capillary beds.

All of these critical components are necessary for developing any muscle quickly and completely. Multi-joint Basic Exercises are important as they hit the majority of muscle fibers in one go.

Stretch Position Exercises are just as important in a muscle-sculpting strength producing program. In fact, stretch position type exercise can accelerate sculpting gains quickly. So for maximum size effects, you should use all of the above. If you train intensely in each of those positions, you ramp up key anabolic hormones threefold.

The Endurance-Component focuses on lighter-to-medium-resistance rather than max force tension. Due to fatigue accumulation within the muscle the Ten By Ten Method requires less tension output. Which is excellent for muscle building hypertrophy within that pathway. The Trainee quickly builds every facet of the muscle and will increase their chiseled muscle and strength gains faster! Plus, you'll add increased vascularity and hard-as-nails-muscle detail, with full-blown pumps at every single workout.

Now for a few comments on the ideal rep speed for muscle growth and strength gains. The best tempo is a 2 second positive and a 2-3 second negative. (Up and Down motion) Why should trainees use this power type tempo to build muscle more efficiently? Two to Three second turnarounds stimulate the power-oriented fibers due to the quick turnaround. This activates significantly more muscle fibers to fire efficiently at a rapid muscle-producing rate.

However, this switch of direction is really a controlled turnaround for the two-second positive at the pre-stretched elongated position. This activates more fast-twitch muscle fibers, which is one reason why the Ten By Ten Method is effective. Once you reach full-range exhaustion, in say the decline pushups, you lower yourself to the stretched position continuing with Ten half reps within the strongest muscle-building- stimulating-point. Controlled half reps of course.

This forces the muscle to continue firing, activating the pre-stretching trigger point getting more dormant endurance fast-twitch fibers into firing at it's maximum. The Best-Time-Under-Tension-Range for strength is about 40 to 50 seconds per set for chiseled muscle-growth-development. The trainee should perform 3-4 exercises. This extends the growth process. Increasing tension time to 2-3 minutes per set for optimum muscle sculpting stimulation.

As stated earlier, this book is geared toward extending the trainee's tension time for chiseled muscle-size instead of just strength gains. So getting into the efficient hypertrophic tension time within 40 to 60 seconds has a lot of potential for triggering loads of new sculpted growth and growth hormone pumping release. Reps between 15 and 30, depending on rep speed, will get you there and stimulate incredible sculpted gains.

CHAPTER 4

The 20, 20, 20, Pre-Stretch-Overload-Muscle-Building Master Plan Plus Change to Grow

Change to Grow: Change to Create Greater Irritation

Years ago while experimenting with enhancing the effects of stretch-position exercises and combining them with the Ten by Ten Method it added another important component which added hardness and enhanced my physique to another level. I thought, I've stumbled upon another method, and it produced such great gains that I need to see how long and what will another 10 weeks produce.

Back then, as I've said earlier in my Bio, I took to the books again. With that, I've realized that in building muscle size, one needs to directly expand sarcoplasm, the muscle energy fluid, as well as thickening of the myofibrils, the strands that are in charge of force-generation. It took some doing but, I soon realized that stretch-position type exercises can build both of those muscle-size components. Stretch position exercises wake up the majority of fibers to fire, including many sleeping dormant endurance fibers.

The reason? The muscle is placed into a full elongation position, then forced to contract forcefully producing a great number of muscle fibers to fire making each contraction far stronger and efficient against it's resistance. With the efficiency of this muscle-producing power of this pre-stretching overload effect, why not tag on a stress method to the most muscle-stimulation position? Along with extended time under tension which will prompt hormone producing pumps.

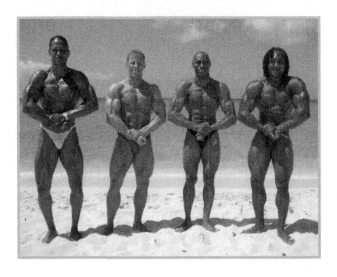

Beyond Self Resistance 85

20, 20, 20 Method

The key to hypertrophic muscle-producing tension time as said before is based on becoming an expert on muscle function, and feel. The best exercises for stimulating the hard to reach fibers are those that have the most stress at the pre-stretched point. All stretch position type exercises fall into that category. I believe that you can make incredible gains using max-stretch resistance type exercises with high reps.

I've experimented with this protocol, and I've attained tremendous results. High-rep pre-stretch-moves first within your workouts, will trigger greater muscle stress on the targeted muscle as well as loosening up muscle casings to promote muscle growth. With this protocol the trainee is stretching against resistance 60 times with a 20-20-20 Method! In the workouts that follow, you start with a high-rep sequence on the stretch position type move, then you do the muscle-teamwork and contracted-type exercises in a 20-20-20 format.

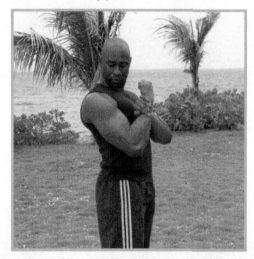

The 20,20,20 method is great for any bodypart including the biceps. Try it out and give it a go.

There's no question that to continue improving your physique, something in your workouts has to change. It's the key to muscle stress adaptation. The trainee must subject their muscles to something new, or they have no reason to improve. My method of developing various stress methods and muscle building hybrids adds strength increases and chiseled muscle development generating more force output on the muscles being worked. Strands in the muscle fibers and connective tissues will thicken. However, the trainee will get stronger with an enhanced neuromuscular efficiency.

Low rep work will not stress the muscle fibers, and will not increase much in muscle size, if at all, with lower-rep strength work. The sarcoplasm is considered to be the major contributor to muscle size. It's a misconception that most trainees think strength gains equal size gains. Continuous change is the answer. Later on in this book I've listed a number of various training modules for the trainee to follow. Which will coax enough muscle-coaxing stimuli that will enhance improvement.

At the bottom of a decline pushup, for example, when you shift direction, there's an extreme pre-stretching overload effect as your chest muscles elongate to the point of pre-stretch and then the trainee reverses the movement. But there's a problem. Most exercises need a reversing turn-around to improve muscle-stimulation efficiency. Other pre-stretching exercises require a pause to promote the best muscle stimulating response.

Key muscle-stimulating-generation is at the half mark point of the exercise stroke. Some below the middle of the exercise motion, at the bottom stretch position of most exercises. Therefore, overloading that position at full stretch, with a pause. You can stimulate the hormonal effects of any rep tremendously! Which means much more growth stimulation and muscle pumps every set.

That's exactly what I did for my contest prep to increase the size and shape of my muscles at every rep. On the pre-stretch it's important to pause for a 3-5 count before reversing the movement per rep. This muscle stretching turnaround promotes the strongest muscle-building signal within that position. Activating a very strong stretch reflex action within the muscle spinals. The partial range of an exercise, is the strongest muscle-building signal within that range of motion. I've cleared up a number of elements so, all the trainee need to do is follow and learn.

An example, take the regular curl for instance one movement pulling all the way up, the other to the mid-point of the exercise stroke. Same exercise movement, same results right? No. Here's the answer: While the hardest part of the movement is the starting position, normally momentum kicks in, making that part of the curl useless. While reducing the stress on the targeted muscle, as well as the finished position, tension drops off of the target muscle. On the other hand pulling the arm to the strongest position of the movement the mid-point, this increases the overload on the muscles amplifying the activity producing a greater muscle building over-load within that position. What is the muscle building trigger?

From turnaround to the strongest muscle building signal produces hypertrophic overload at the strongest stimulating spot within that key exercise stroke. The trainee receives extreme hormonal overload within that range of motion. This overloads the endurance-oriented-fast-twitch fibers at the precise muscle stimulating point to create greater muscle overload within that position, exactly where the muscle needs it the most. Yes, there are two points along the exercise's stroke, but—and this is key—not at the point of maximum contraction, The spot in the range that is the main hypertrophic growth response.

The mid-point and turnaround point is where it is at—where the body changes directions—is one of the key spot for most exercises. It's where maximum force is generated by the target muscles.

These two points on certain exercises are where extreme overload takes place for extreme muscle fiber stimulation. For years I've heard the same old full range of motion, will increase flexibility, muscle size and strength.
However, a more effective and efficient form of training is to overload the semi-stretch point at the end of full reps by activating the stretch reflex position at each rep... Standard full reps are good—but they're slow growth producers.

Why? Two reasons.

Reason One: One is that you can't generate nearly enough force to trigger much growth stimulation during normal full reps, no matter how many reps you do. The trainee will never overload the muscles enough to create enough irritation to promote a steady growth process.

Reason Two: Even if the trainee do sets to positive failure, the trainee will receive limited hormonal stimulation because the trainee's nervous system gets fried before their muscles do. That's right, your nervous system stops you right when you're starting to activate the key endurance oriented fast-twitch growth fibers. Is it necessary for a trainee to perform set after set of exercises? So you, the trainee may eventually get some growth stimuli, but at what cost? You burn up so much energy and recovery ability that growth will never happen, or at least it becomes very difficult.

In short the trainee becomes over-trained. This is not an efficient way to stimulate any form of muscle growth or strength. That's the reason why so many self resistance practitioners receive miniscule amounts of progress. Due to overuse and not activating the important endurance fibers.
Think about it. This book was developed to clear up the many misconceptions on self resistance training and how to efficiently get the most out of every single rep and set.

There is a correlation between muscle burn and growth hormone release. Within this book the trainee will learn how to scorch the target muscle that's being trained. Blood-flow blockage, along with various hybrid stress methods place undue irritation and stress onto the trained muscle, to promote strength and muscle growth.

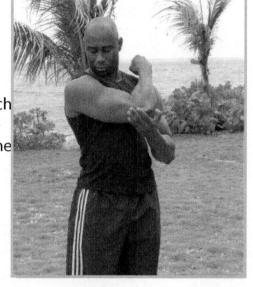

That's the reason size-building effectiveness takes place due to various stress methods which activates an abundance of muscle-fiber activation—a serious growth hormone surge from the muscle burn. Plus, by tacking them on to the muscle-teamwork exercises, like decline push-ups or, three chair dips the trainee increases their testosterone levels production threefold. Multi-joint Teamwork exercises are key for increasing testosterone production).

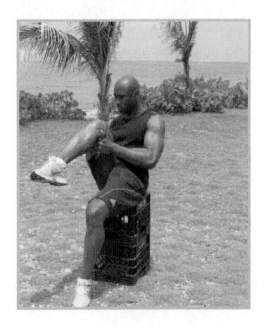

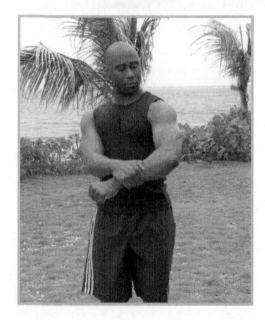

Chapter 5

The
Ideal Rep Speed
for
Chiseled Growth plus Enhancing
Beyond Growth Enhancing
Super-Pumps
with
Muscle Building lessons

The Ideal Rep Speed for Chiseled Growth

As before, The best rep speed for chiseled muscle development and strength is a two-three second positive and a two-three-second negative—In short up and down phase. Using a power cadence, which is one second up and one second down. Produce some serious strength gains within the musculature being trained.

This faster rep speed suggestion (power cadence) causes extreme damage to more muscle fibers than slower traditional rep speeds. So what is the key? It's, the forceful reversed turnaround for the one-to-two-second positive and negative movement. That explosive jolt right at the semi-stretch stage of the targeted muscle activates significantly more muscle fibers, which force the muscle to continue firing, activating the stretch reflex and getting more dormant fibers into firing.

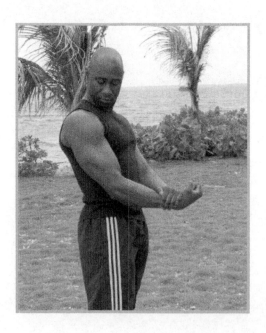 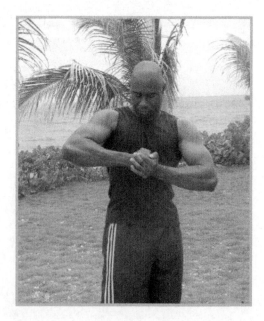

Muscle-Building Lesson 1: The pre-stretched point of an exercise's stroke is key. You need to overload the strongest muscle-building range, especially on the turnaround point of any exercise, if you want to maximize your muscle-sculpting gains. The best way is with power-point-reps at the end of a set, or within the set which are a series of partial reps right off the bat that encompasses the semi-stretched position, along with, various hybrid methods on almost every exercise within this muscle-sculpting-building course. I will review and analyze the stress-method-techniques, later in this book.

Let's get down into the training effects of continuous-tension exercises. They are important because they block blood flow to the targeted muscle being trained. Occlusion is the name of the game here. So, why does blocking blood flow produce such spectacular increases in muscle? Part of it may be due to the influx of blood to the body part. Increasing the capillary network within the muscle structure walls.

The most beneficial part of your training is at the very ending of the set. That is where most occlusion is occurring. However, what normally happens most? — You stop your set short. So by, terminating the set too soon you the trainee are robbing yourself of some extra-muscle-coaxing and strength increases. From experience I've developed a method of doing continuous-tension exercises to increase neuromuscular efficiency.

This keeps the muscle firing as more occlusion occurs. Even though the pain you will receive while performing your reps will indeed hurt, hang in there for it's the last few reps that count. However, with stress methods and various hybrid-expanded stress methods you will skip ahead of the static response early, by stimulating and enhancing fiber-recruitment. That's where efficiency of effort comes in. So the trainee progresses at a faster rate.

Training a little smarter is what this book is about. It is designed to show and teach the trainee, how to keep enough tension on the targeted muscles for full occlusion to occur. This enhances the anabolic effects even further. For greater chiseled hard muscle and strength gains. The stress methods and routines force the muscle to contract harder without using maximum tension, keeping muscle-stimulating tension on the muscles instead of the joints.

The importance of the pump is very important with your training, and every trainee should aim to achieve it. Continuous tension reps increases the surge of not only occlusion (blood blockage), it creates loads of hormonal surges to take place within the system. Increasing strength and enhancing muscle building power. Not only that but, within this book, there are loads of precise details and warm up variables to enhance muscle chiseled growth.

Muscle-Building Lesson 2: It is important to increase force-production at the pre-stretched position on every exercise, the trainee's quest should be to strive for continuous tension for massive blood blockage. There will be phases where there is a isolation exercise before, or after and even combined (superset) with basic exercises to enhance the muscle building response threefold. This produces concentrated continuous tension, with significant blood-blockage impairment, which in turn stimulates another level of muscle growth.

Special Note: Most isolation exercises will be performed at the mid-point of the exercise stroke to occlude the muscle properly. An example would be resisted forward raises that hits the bottom two-thirds of the exercise of each rep to maintain continuous tension.

CHAPTER 6

Increasing Hormonal Surges
and
Fiber Overload

Increasing Hormonal Surges and Fiber Overload

I've been asked several times, what exercises produce the best growth response? The body's muscular structures work best as a single unit as opposed to a sum of parts. Meaning, it's best for a group of muscles work together, instead of separated. Once the muscle structures work together they produce maximum force production for greater muscle overload. Which increases Growth Hormone and testosterone production.

Those are the reasons I have included a combination of synergy (Basic-Muscle-Teamwork) exercises within the workout plans. As mentioned in the last chapter, isolation type exercises for occlusion is needed for increased muscle burn. The muscle-burn is directly linked to growth hormone release. Due to higher blood lactic acid levels, that is partially responsible for muscle burn, along with the blood-blockage effect.

Why is ramping Growth hormone and testosterone surges important? It creates an amazing growth environment. So, including basic and isolation (blood-block-age) exercises this isolates the stress on the musculature and keeps the pressure on the muscles being worked, creating a bigger pump. So, am I really saying basic exercises alone within a program are inferior by themselves?

From a (blood-blockage) standpoint: yes. It is also inferior in terms of occlusion and keeping the tension on the working muscles. For basic (muscle-team work) exercises stimulate the target muscle at most times ¼ or ½ mark within the movement and tension drops off after that. However, there are ways to get more irritation on the muscles with basic exercises by including stress methods to enhance the muscle burn for occlusion within the muscle's structures.

Fiber Overload

Taking your basic exercises and applying power partials, or stress methods at certain positions at various exercises. An example: on regular curls, perform all your full reps, followed by partial power reps from the bottom position to the mid-point. This will increase force production and the trainee's biceps will get far stronger with the increased force of contraction and blood blockage.
The exercise method works even better at a fully pre-stretched position like decline pushups.

By extending your set further, move to the bottom position of the exercise at the (reverse position), and perform the power partial stress method to failure. An extreme pre-stretch within that position will loosen up the fibers and growth potential to greater muscle pumping proportions. Now, genetics has a lot to do with how much growth potential the muscle has, so your attention to precision and tremendous effort with pre-stretched-position exercises are key.

In my earlier experiments I learned to overload my chest in the stretched position with partial rep decline pushups. I did this at the bottom-stretched position to the midpoint only, then reversed the movement. This increased the occlusion effect via continuous tension, which irritates the chest muscles with extreme stretch overload, along with creating increased fiber splitting—which in turn means the more fibers you have, the bigger your muscles can become!

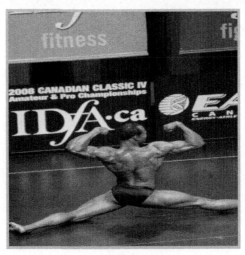

Muscle-building lesson 3: While pre-stretching and overloading the muscles is important, it is important that the trainee understand that stretch-position type exercises trigger hormonal activation within the muscles that, trigger increased fiber activation. It's growth producing factors that can get you chiseled at a faster rate! (There will be loads of stretch-position type exercises for each body part later in this book along with the Double- Dip Stress method).

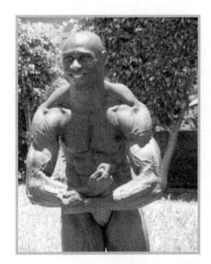 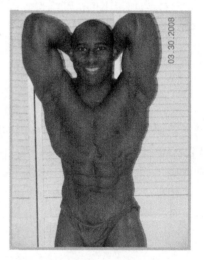

Marlon continues to prgress with the help of Hybrid Methods.

Chapter 7

Increasing Neuromuscular Efficiency by Covering the Angles

What is the best way to increase your neuromuscular efficiency? The best way to activate the motor-unit effect to increase more fast-twitch fibers, is to add a few sets with Stress Methods tagged onto your sets before the nervous system shut-down. That way, there is no nervous system fatigue and you keep the key endurance oriented fast twitch fibers firing right at the key point of the exercise stroke.

My hybrid stress method strategy will make each set five times more effective than standard reps and sets. Using a variety of different exercises can stimulate different muscle fibers. Multi-angular strength producing exercises stimulates more fibers to fire at different ranges of push and pull. Changing the pull or push position, changes muscle fiber recruitment patterns.

The order of muscle fiber recruitment can also change for multifunctional muscles from one movement or exercise to another. Recruitment order in the Upper-back for pull-downs are different from that of a across the body pull. In order to fully recruit various muscle fibers, and to completely develop a particular muscle, it must be exercised with several exercises."

Muscle-building lesson 4: You must train a muscle from various angles— in order to stimulate efficient fiber activation. Most exercises fall between basic, pre-stretch and contracted position type categories, with an added Stress-Method or hybrid techniques, which I will explain later in various chapters. This creates a serious muscle-stimulating irritation that stimulates a very quick growth response!

Unless you've read Beyond 15 Week Mini Course Workout 1/or tried the Stress Rep techniques, you may not realize just how powerful it is. Most times, at the very end of the set, when the muscles are fatigued the trainee stops the set too soon. Preventing the trainee from reaching his or her ultimate goal. That's right, the set stops before the important growth-producing reps kick in, and so muscle growth stimulation is to a bare minimum.

But with Stress Methods, instead of stopping, you perform various partial power-point reps at the strongest muscle-building-point. That is the only way a trainee can really stimulate and recruit the endurance-oriented-fast-twitch fibers. Getting more fast-twitch-fiber involvement with efficient training is only part of the Stress Method's extraordinary power. However, there is the occlusion element as well, because stress techniques and methods create enough continuous tension, occlusion and hormonal output within the set to create a massive muscle-stimulating effect.

As I mentioned earlier, most trainees stop their sets too early to fully reap all the strength-building benefits of time under tension, and time under load, which will create longer occlusion times and your muscle sculpting gains will skyrocket to greater heights. As well as, enhancing neuromuscular efficiency. Stress techniques and methods can help you overcome that limitation of poor muscle-to-nerve pathways to greater neuromuscular efficiency output.

As the trainee, you will realize stress methods power partials at various muscle producing points increases force-production at the strongest muscle stimulating spot. Hence, the blockage of blood flow for increased pumps and occlusion-muscle-growth effects— once there's occlusion, there's usually burn. That my friend is the growth hormone efficiency of training.

Performing Stress Methods to any set can trigger an intense muscle burn at will—on just about any exercise. That means you create a greater surge of GH release and testosterone secretions within the muscle for enhanced anabolic surges. Stress Methods produce spectacular muscle-sculpting and hardening results, as the gains I made in a matter of a few months of training in '2008.

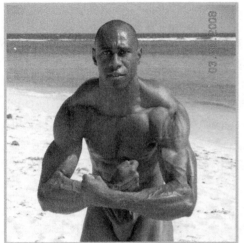 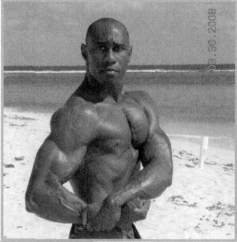

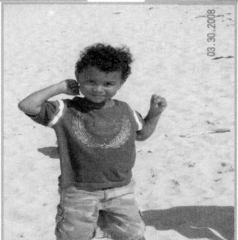

Not only was I getting ready to compete, young Kai gave instructions as well.

"Stress Methods are the single most efficient muscle-producing concept to come along in years." However, there's more — I've even developed various, hybrid techniques that can take the trainee to greater levels.

Contest Day April 2008 the Difference between March and April

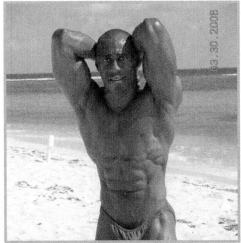
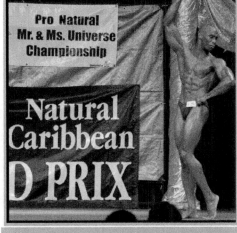
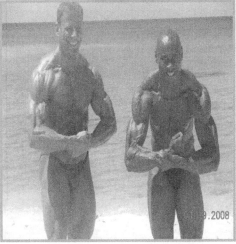
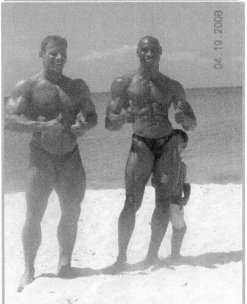

Marlon show time top right 1.3% Bodyfat. Along with, the after show photoshoot. What fun. Even young Kai had a part in the events.

Muscle-building lesson 5: Change on a regular basis can create faster adaptation, i.e. growth and strength gains. That's the reason you need a variety of Stress-Method-Hybrid techniques in your mass-stimulating program. Switch the methods up every 3-4 weeks so full adaptation doesn't occur often. This will provide your muscles with greater stress overload to coax a greater muscle building stimuli.

Muscle-Building Lessons Review

Lesson 1: The pre-stretched point of an exercise is vital. It is important to overload the strongest muscle-building position if you want to maximize your gains.

Lesson 2: Strive for continuous tension to block blood flow on at least all muscle-stimulating exercises. It's a great reason to use isolation exercises either before, or after the basic multi-joint type exercises for enhanced—concentrated continuous tension.

Lesson 3: While pre-stretching and continuous tension are important, take note that, stretch-position type exercises ramp up anabolic hormones and trigger greater fiber splitting effects. It's another layer of growth production that can get the muscles stronger and more chiseled much faster!New Hybrid Double-Dip tactic on stretch-position exercises supercharge muscle-stimulating-gains.

Lesson 4: You must train a muscle from a variety of angles— of push and pull in order to efficiently enhance muscle fiber activation. Add Stress Methods and advanced hybrid techniques, to each position to maximize size stimulation faster than before!

Lesson 5: Change on a regular basis to avoid adaptation. Vary the Stress-Methods and Hybrid techniques every 3-4 weeks in a phase approach. For once the body fully adapts progress stops.

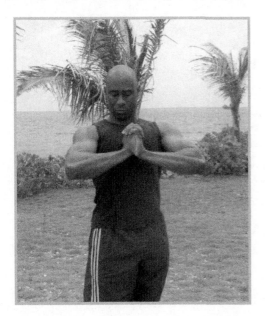 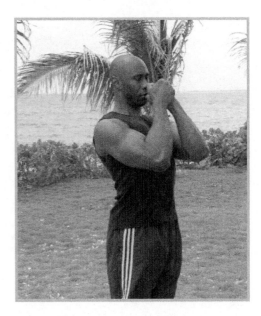

Take a look at Marlon's muscularity in his shoulder, forearms and triceps. Now, That's efficiency of effort, with solid science to bodybuilding.

CHAPTER 8

20,20,20
Hybrid Stress Method
is Born

20,20,20 Hybrid Stress Method

After various experiments with Stress-Methods I tried other hybrid methods to see what type of training effect it would produce. So, I started off at the strongest muscle building spot. This was performed from the pre-stretched position up to the midpoint for reps of 20. This was followed by another 20 full range reps straight off the bat, and then a last 20 at the fully stretched position to mid-point.

This hybrid method increased my physique threefold and I noticed each time I tried the method within a 3 week phase, it created a sudden jolt of hard chiseled muscularity and increased vascularity. This technique I realized was a very unique way of ramping new stress-overload on the musculature! The 20,20,20 Hybrid Method was born.

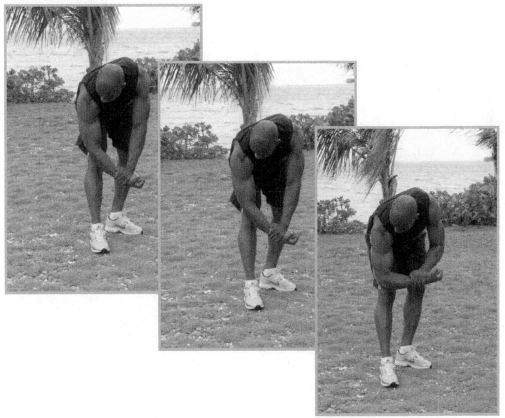

This hybrid method overload the pre-stretched elongated position at the get go. Creating extreme anabolic reactions within the position. Due to the blood-blockage effect, the 20,20,20 Stress Method, causes the endurance fast-twitch fibers to fire efficiently without overbearing tendon and ligament support.

The spectacular size and strength increases from the 20,20,20 method blew my mind. Combining power partial reps at the strongest muscle building position first with a semi-stretch is the most important point in many exercises near the turnaround position.

Shifting from the bottom pre-stretched position to the strongest muscle-stimulating signal. This overloads the muscle to fire harder due to the reversing of the turnaround point of the exercise stroke. Combining that with full reps and again hitting that important stroke again within the reverse position increases growth threefold.

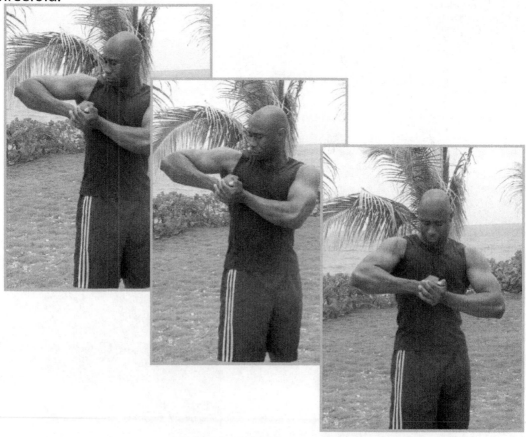

How does that cause more muscle growth? Excessive overload at the strongest muscle-stimulating position is the key fiber-activation point on the exercise position, which is the mid-point. At this position maximum force production will occur. This will allow the trainee to achieve more target-muscle overload, straight off the bat.

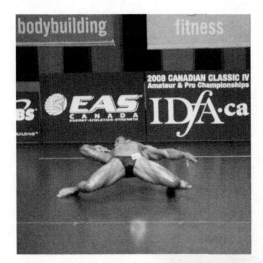
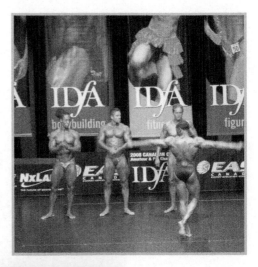

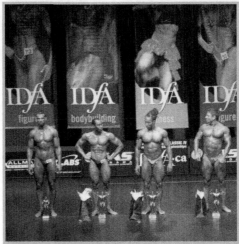

Marlon demontrating his flexibility and balance within his routine.

CHAPTER 9

20,20, 20
Hybrid Stress Method
Phase One

20,20,20 Hybrid Stress Method

20,20, 20 HYBRID STRESS METHOD PHASE ONE 3 weeks

* Remember with this method you perform 20 reps at the start to mid point, followed by 20 full reps, and to finish off 20 reps at the start to mid point again, Then rest. Alternate Day One and Day Two for 6 days of training. 3 sets per exercise
Day One

LEGS
Stiff legged press (full reps)
*Crossed feet squats
*Resisted leg extension
*Resisted leg curls

CALVES
Slanted calve raises (full reps)
Standing calve raises (full reps)

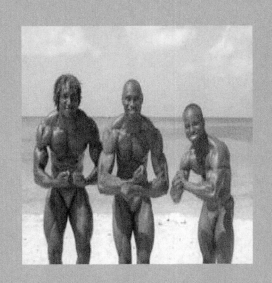

UPPER CHEST
*Decline pushups
 Upper chest press (full reps)

LOWER CHEST
*Three chair pushups
Liederman press (full reps)

TRICEPS
*Over head tricep press
*Forward lateral press
*Tricep pressdown

 FOREARMS
 Palm up wrist curls (full reps)
 Palm down wrist curls (full reps)
 Forearm press (full reps)

Day Two

UPPERBACK
*Three chair dips
* Resisted pulldowns
* Stiff arm pulldown

UPPER TRAPS
Front neck press (full reps)
Side to side press (full reps)
Rear neck press   (full reps)

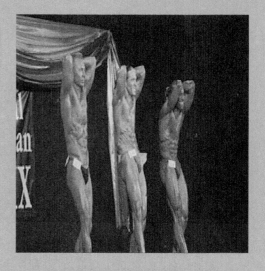

SHOULDERS

Across the body lateral raises (full reps)
*Decline pushups
*Resisted forward raises
Across the body pulls (full reps)

BICEPS
*Palm up curls
*Hammer curls
*Reverse curls
*Concentration curls

Abs
Reverse crunches (full reps)

CHAPTER 9

20,20, 20
Hybrid Stress Method
Phase Two

PHASE TWO   3 WEEKS

Day One

LOWER CHEST
* Three chair pushups
Liederman press (full reps)

UPPER CHEST
*Decline pushups
 Upper chest press (full reps)

TRICEPS
 *Over head tricep press
 *Tricep pressdown
 * Forward lateral press
  Decline tricep press

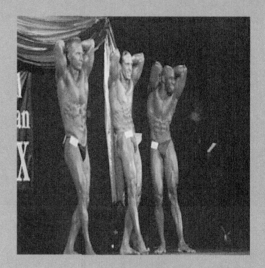

Day Two

CALVES
Slanted calve raises (full reps)
Standing calve raises (full reps)

LEGS
*Crossed leg squats
*One legged squats (optional)
*Resisted leg extension (optional)
 Stiff legged press (full reps)
*Resisted leg curls

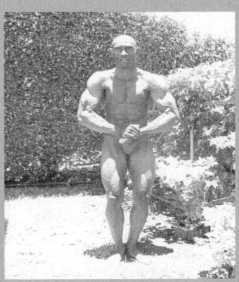

UPPER TRAPS
Side to side neck press (full reps)
Behind the back pull (full reps)
Rear neck presses (full reps)

ABS
Reverse crunches (full reps)
Across the body situps (full reps)
Across the body side crunches (full reps)

Day Three

UPPERBACK
*Three chair dips
*Thigh rows (full reps)

Mid-Traps
Across the body rows (full reps)
Behind the back pulls (full reps)

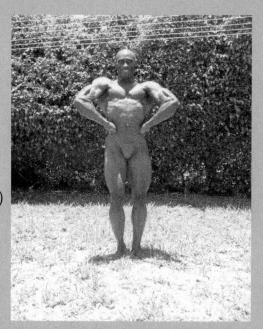

UPPER TRAPS
Forward neck press (full reps)
Rear neck press (full reps)

SHOULDERS
Across the body lateral raises (full reps)
Across the body pulls (full reps)
*Decline pushups
* Resisted forward raises

BICEPS
*Palm up curls
*Over head bicep curls
*Resisted concentration curls

FOREARMS
*Reverse curls
*Hammer curls
Forearm press
Palm down reverse wrist curls

Perform day one,two and three. Then, repeat day one again. Train on this phase for 6 days a week.

CHAPTER 10

Ten by Ten
Hybrid Stress Method
Phase One

TEN BY TEN METHOD
PHASE ONE 3 weeks

Within this routine the trainee performs 10 full reps, followed by 10 half reps. From the start position to mid-point. If 10 by 10 is too easy increase the reps to 15 by 15. On the third day start again at day one and continue with the program. 6 days a week of training. 3 Sets per exercise.

Day One

UPPER TRAPS
Rear neck press (full reps)
Side to side press (full reps)

UPPERBACK
*Resisted pulldowns
*Three chair dips
Thigh rows (full reps)

SHOULDERS
*Decline pushups
 Across the body lateral raises (full reps)
*Resisted forward raises
 Across the body pulls (full reps)

BICEPS
*Palm up curls
*Hammer curls
*Overhead curls
*Concentration curls

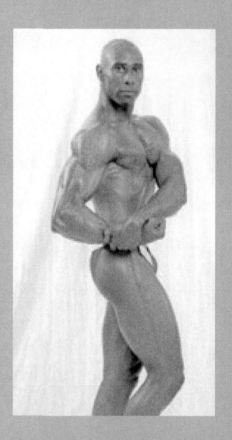

Day Two

LEGS
*One legged squats
*Resisted leg extensions
*Resisted leg curls

CALVES
*Slanted calve raises
*Standing calve raises

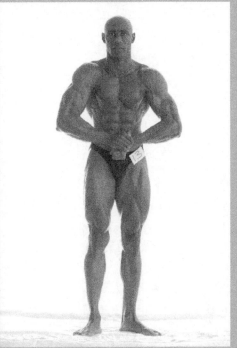

LOWER BACK/HAMSTRINGS
Stiff legged press (full reps)

UPPER TRAPS
Rear neck press (full reps)
Side to side neck press (full reps)
Behind the back pulls (full reps)

FOREARMS
Palm up wrist curls (full reps)
Palm down reverse wrist curls (full reps)
*Reverse curls

Day Three

UPPER CHEST
*Decline pushups
*Upper chest press

LOWER CHEST
*Three chair pushups
*Decline pushups
 Liederman press (full reps)

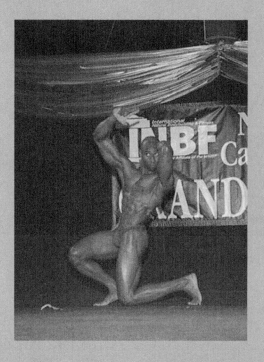

TRICEPS
*Palm up tricep pressdown
*Overhead tricep press
*Forward lateral press
 Decline tricep extension (full reps)

ABS
Reverse crunches (full reps)

CHAPTER 10

Ten by Ten Hybrid
Stress Method
Phase Two

Ten by Ten Hybrid Stress Method

PHASE TWO

Perform this routine for 6 days straight. Alternating day one and day two for another 3 weeks. 3 Sets per exercise.

Day One
UPPER CHEST
*Decline pushups

LOWER CHEST
*Three chair pushups
Liederman press (full reps)

UPPER BACK
Thigh rows (full reps)
*Stiff arm pulldown
Across the body rows (full reps)

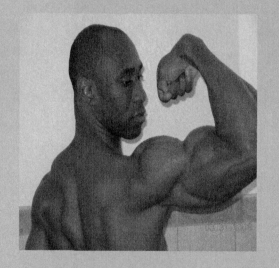

UPPER TRAPS
Rear neck press (full reps)
Side to side neck press (full reps)
Behind the back pulls (full reps)

BICEPS
*Reverse curls
*Hammer curls
*Concentration curls

CALVES
*Standing calve raises

FOREARMS
Reverse palm down wrist curls (full reps)
Palm up wrist curls (full reps)

DAY TWO
UPPER TRAPS
Side to side neck press (full reps)
Rear neck press (full reps)
Forward neck press (full reps)

SHOULDERS
*Resisted forward raises
*Across the body lateral raises
*Resisted forward raises
 Across the body pulls

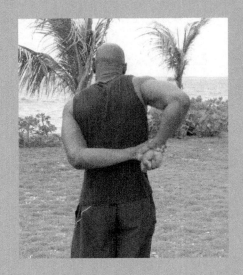

TRICEPS
Decline pushups (full reps)
*Overhead tricep press
*Tricep pressdown
*Forward lateral press

LEGS
*One legged squats
*leg extensions
* leg curls

CALVES
*Standing calve raises
*Slanted calve raises

FOREARMS
Forearm press (full reps)
*Reverse curls
*Hammer curls
 Reverse wrist curls palm down

CHAPTER 11

Double Impact
Hybrid Stress Method
Phase One

DOUBLE IMPACT
PHASE ONE 3 WEEKS

Perform this method by alternating a full rep and a half rep. Every full and half rep is one rep. Only exercises with an * will be perform in double impact style. Perform 3 sets each exercise. 6 Days per week training.

Day One
CHEST
*Decline pushups
*Three chair pushups
Liederman press

UPPER BACK
*Three chair dips
* Stiff arm pulldowns
Across the body rows

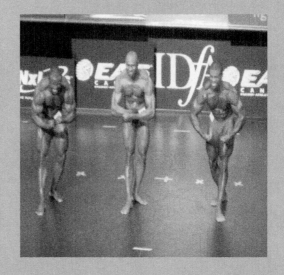

BICEPS
*Palm up curls
*Reverse curl
*Hammer curl
*Overhead curl

CALVES
*Standing calve raises
*Slanted calve raises

Double Impact Hybrid Stress Method

Day Two
UPPER TRAPS
Rear neck press (full reps)
Forward neck press (full reps)
Resisted upright pulls

SHOULDERS
* Forward raises
* Across the body lateral raises
* Decline pushups
  Across the body pulls (full reps)

 TRICEPS
 * Forward lateral press
 * Tricep pressdown
 * Palm up tricep pressdown
 * Overhead tricep press

LEGS
*One legged squats
* Crossed feet squats
* leg extensions
* leg curls

CALVES
*Standing calve raises
* slanted calve raises

ABS
Reverse crunches (full reps) 30

FOREARMS
Forearm press (full reps)
Reverse wrist curls (full reps)
Palm up wrist curls (full reps)

CHAPTER 11

Double Impact Hybrid
Stress Method
Phase Two

PHASE TWO 3 WEEKS (SUPERSET)

Supersets are two exercises done back to back then the trainee rest and
repeat for 3 sets. Alternate day one and day two for 6 days of training.
An * states the double impact method applied to the exercise.
On supersets perform all reps on one side both movements then switch sides.

Day One
CHEST
Liederman press
* Decline pushups (superset)

*Three chair pushups
Liederman press (superset)

UPPERBACK
Across the body rows (full reps)
Across the body pulls (full reps) (superset)

*Stiff arm pulldowns
*Three chair dips

UPPER TRAPS
Rear neck press (full reps)
Side to side neck press (full reps) (superset)

BICEPS
* Palm up curls
* Overhead curls (superset)

Routine Continued......

BICEPS
*Palm up curl
* Reverse curl (superset)

*Concentration curls

CALVES
Slanted calve raises
Standing calve raises (superset)

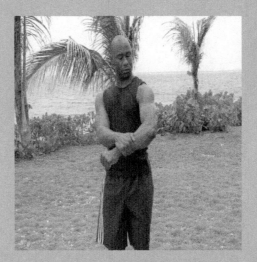

Day Two

UPPER TRAPS
Rear neck press (full reps)
Forward neck press (full reps) (superset)

Side to side neck press (full reps)
Rear neck press (full reps) (superset)

SHOULDERS
Resisted upright pulls (full reps)
*Resisted shoulder press (superset)

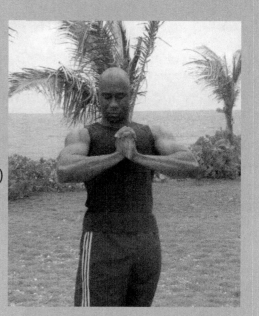

*Forward raises
* Across the body lateral raises (superset)

Across the body pulls (full reps)

TRICEPS
 *Palm up pressdown
* Forward lateral press (superset)

*Overhead tricep press
* Forward lateral press (superset)

Routine Continued......

LEGS
* One legged squats
* Leg extensions (superset)

Stiff legged press
*Leg curls

CALVES
Standing calve raises
Slanted calve raises (superset)

FOREARMS
Palm up wrist curls
Reverse palm down wrist curls (superset)

*Reverse curls
*Hammer curls (superset)

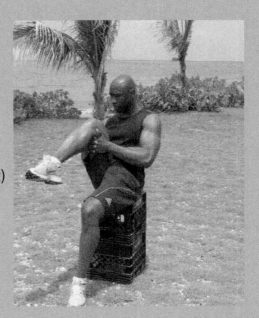

CHAPTER 12

Compound Isolation Hybrid Stress Method Phase One

COMPOND ISOLATION Routine
PHASE ONE 3 WEEKS

Remember with this method the trainee will perform one exercise by itself, then superset two exercises. An * states superset the two exercises. 3 Sets each exercise, at 15-20 reps each movement.

DAY ONE
CHEST
Decline pushups

*Decline pushups
*Liederman press (superset)

*Three chair pushups
*Upper chest press (superset)

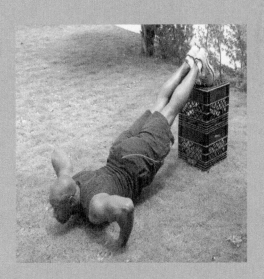

 UPPER BACK
 Three chair dips

*Across the body rows
*Across the body pulls (superset)

*Thigh rows
*Stiff arm pulldowns (superset)

Routine Continued..........

UPPER TRAPS
Side to side neck press

*Rear neck press
*Forward neck press (superset)

BICEPS
Palm up curls

*Palm up curls
*Overhead bicep curls (superset)

Concentration curls
FOREARMS

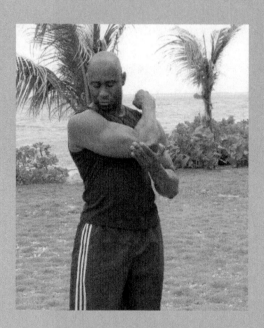

*Reverse curls
*Hammer curls (superset)

*Palm up wrist curls
*Palm down wrist curls (superset)

CALVES
Standing calve raises

*Slanted calve raises
*Standing calve raises (superset)

DAY TWO

UPPER TRAPS
Resisted upright pulls

*Side to side neck press
*Rear neck press (superset)

LEGS
One legged squats

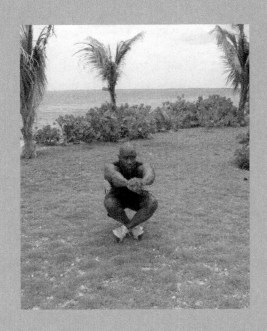

*One legged squats
*Leg extensions (superset)

Leg curls
Stiff legged press

UPPER/LOWER BACK
Thigh rows

SHOULDERS
Resisted shoulder press

*Across the body lateral raises
* Forward raises (superset)

*Resisted upright pulls
*Behind the back pulls (superset)

*Forward raises
*Across the body pulls (superset)

Routine Continued.........

TRICEPS
Decline tricep extensions

*Overhead tricep press
*Forward lateral press (superset)

*Overhead tricep press
*Tricep pressdown (superset) (palm up or regular)

FOREARMS
Reverse curls

*Palm down wrist curls
*Hammer curls (superset)

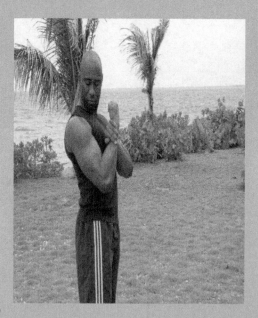

CALVES
*Slanted calve raises
*Standing calves raises (superset)

ABS
Reverse crunches

*Reverse crunches
* Across the body crunches (superset)

CHAPTER 12

Compound Isolation
Hybrid Stress Method
Phase Two

Compound Isolation Hybrid Stress Method

PHASE TWO Slightly different than Phase One. The Trainee will Perform Three exercises together as a Tri-set, then rest. Same 3 sets of each exercise at 15-20 reps. 6 Days of training for 3 weeks.

DAY ONE
CHEST
*Decline pushups
*Liederman press
*Upper chest press (tri-set)

 UPPER TRAPS
*Side to side neck press
*Rear neck press
*Forward neck press (tri-set)

 UPPERBACK
*Resisted pulldowns
*Stiff arm pulldown
*Three chair dips (tri-set)

UPPER/LOWER BACK
Thigh rows

 BICEPS
*Palm up curl
*Hammer curl
*Concentration curl (tri-set)

Routine Continued........

FOREARMS
*Palm down reverse wrist curls
*Palm up wrist curls
*Forearm press (tri-set)

CALVES
*Slanted calve raises
*Standing calve raises
*Slanted calve raises (tri-set)

ABS
*Reverse crunches
*Across the body crunches
*Reverse crunches (tri-set)

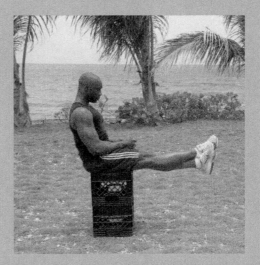

DAY TWO
UPPER TRAPS
*Behind the back pulls
*Resisted upright pulls
*Rear neck press (tri-set)

SHOULDERS
*Resisted forward raises
*Across the body lateral raises
*Resisted shoulder press (tri-set)

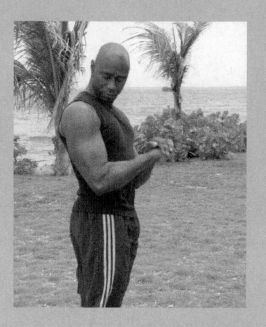

TRICEPS
*Overhead tricep press
*Tricep pressdown
*Forward lateral press (tri-set)

LEGS
*One legged squats
*Leg extensions
*One legged squats (triset)

*Stiff legged press
*Leg curl
*Crossed feet squats (tri-set)

CALVES
*Standing calve raises
*Slanted calve raises
*Standing calve raises (tri-set)

ABS
Reverse crunches

CHAPTER 13

Fiber Overload Hybrid Stress Method Phase One

FIBER OVERLOAD METHOD

Perform this method at the Strongest-Muscle-Building-Signal, the power Point. Or, Mid-Point of the exercise stroke. Training at the half point only. 6 days a week training, 3 sets per exercise at 15 reps each movement. Perform routine for 3 weeks

PHASE ONE
DAY ONE

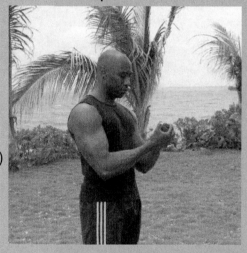

CHEST
Decline pushups (bottom range)
Three chair pushups (bottom range)

UPPER BACK
Three chair dips (bottom range)
Stiff arm pulldowns (top range)

BICEPS
Palm up curl (bottom range)
Reverse curl (bottom range)
Concentration curls (bottom range)

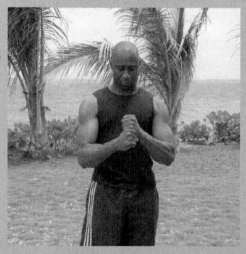

Routine Continued.......

TRICEPS
Triceps pressdowns (start to mid point)
Forward lateral press (start to mid point)
Overhead tricep press (bottom to mid point)

CALVES
Standing calve raises (full reps)
Slanted calve raises (full reps)

UPPER TRAPS
Behind the back pulls (full reps)
Rear neck press (full reps)
Side to side neck press (full reps)

FOREARMS
Palm down reverse wrist curls (full reps)
Palm up wrist curls (full reps)

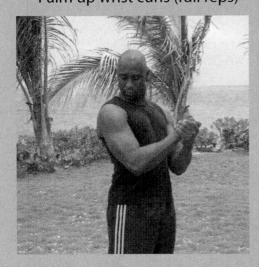 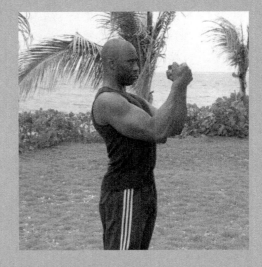

DAY TWO

UPPER TRAPS
Forward neck press (full reps)
Side to side neck press (full reps)

SHOULDERS
Across the body lateral raises (bottom range)
Across the body pulls (full reps)
Resisted forward raises (bottom range)
Decline pushups (elbows out) (bottom range)

LEGS
One legged squats (bottom range)
Crossed feet squats (bottom range)
Leg curls (full reps)
Slanted calve raises (full reps)
Standing calve raises (full reps)

FOREARMS
Hammer curls (bottom range)
Reverse curls   (bottom range)
Palm down reverse wrist curls (full reps)

TRICEPS
Overhead press (full reps)
Palm up tricep pressdown (start to mid point)
Forward lateral press (start to mid point)

ABS
Reverse crunches (full reps)

CHAPTER 13

Fiber Overload Hybrid
Stress Method
Phase Two

PHASE TWO
Within this Phase a combination of Full range of motion exercises will be supersetted with half movements. 3 sets each exercise at 20 reps each exercise .Perform this routine every-other-day for 3 weeks.

WORKOUT ONE

LEGS
*One legged squats (alternate legs) (bottom range)
*Crossed legged squats (superset) (bottom range)

*Leg curls (bottom range)
*Stiff legged press (superset) (full range)

CHEST
*Liederman press (full range)
*Decline pushups (superset) (bottom range)

CHEST
*Three chair pushups (bottom range)
*Upper chest press (superset) (full reps)

UPPERBACK
Thigh rows (full range)
Across the body rows (full reps)

Routine Continued.........

UPPERBACK
*Across the body pulls (full reps)
*Three chair dips (superset) (bottom range)

BICEPS
*Palm up curls (bottom range)
*Reverse curls (superset) (bottom range)

BICEPS
*Hammer curls (bottom range)
*Concentration curls (superset) (bottom range)

TRICEPS
Decline tricep extensions (full reps)

*Overhead tricep press (bottom range)
*Forward lateral tricep press (superset) (start to mid point)

FOREARMS
*Reverse palm down wrist curls (full reps)
*Palm up wrist curls (superset) (full reps)

FOREARMS
*Reverse curls (bottom range)
*Hammer curls (superset) (bottom range)

CHAPTER 14

Double Dip Hybrid
Stress Method

DOUBLE DIP

Perform this stress method at the fully stretched position performing two partial (half) reps followed by a full rep. 3 sets each exercise at 15 reps each. * indicates the exercises used for the double dip method. (Two half reps and one full rep) equals one rep. Perform this routine for 3 WEEKS

Bottom Range… Starting position to mid-point. In some cases like the squat and pushups, it will be the bottom position to mid-point.

Top Range…. Start position to mid-point. An example, resisted pulldowns, Are to be performed from the top position to mid-point.

DAY ONE

UPPER TRAPS
Rear neck press (full reps)
Side to side neck press (full reps)
Behind the back pulls (full reps)

SHOULDERS
*Forward raises (bottom range)
*Decline pushups (elbows out) (bottom range)
  Across the body pulls (full reps)

TRICEPS
*Overhead tricep presses (bottom range to mid-point)
*Forward lateral press (start to midpoint)
*Tricep pressdown (bottom range)

Routine Continued.......

BICEPS
Overhead curls (full range)
*Palm up bicep curl (bottom range)
*Concentration curls (bottom range)
*Reverse curls (bottom range)

CALVES
Standing calve raises (full range)
Slanted calve raises (full range)

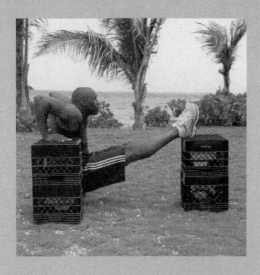 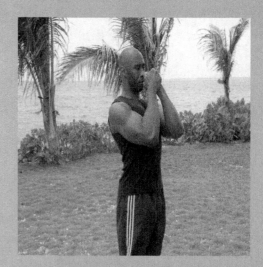

DAY TWO

UPPER BACK
Thigh rows (full range)
*Stiff arm pulldown (top range)
*Resisted pulldowns (top range)
*Three chair dips (bottom range)

CHEST
*Decline pushups (bottom range)
*Three chair pushups (bottom range)
Liederman press (full range)
Upper chest press (full range)

UPPER TRAPS
Rear neck press (full range)
Resisted upright pulls (full range)

LEGS
Stiff legged press (full range)
*Leg curls (bottom range)
*One legged or cross legged squats (bottom range)

CALVES
Standing calve raises (full reps)

ABS
Reverse crunches (full range)

CHAPTER 15

The Original Phase One
Workout
The Beginning
Phase One

THE ORIGINAL PHASE ONE WORKOUT
Perform this routine for 4 weeks full reps only

Day One

Decline Pushups
Liederman Presses
Crossed feet squats
Resisted leg extensions
Leg curls
Resisted pulldowns
Three chair dips
Across the body rows
Decline pushups (elbows out)
Resisted shoulder press
Resisted upright pulls

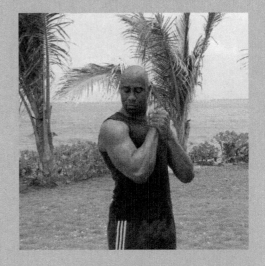

Day Two

Thigh rows
Standing calve raises
Reverse crunches
Across the body side crunches
Resisted forward tricep presses
Tricep pressdown
Bicep curl palm up
Reverse curls
Palm up wrist curls
Palm down wrist curls

The Original Phase One Workout

Day Three

Crossed feet squats
Resisted leg extensions
Resisted leg curls
Standing calve raises
Decline pushups
Liederman presses
Resisted pulldown
Across the body rows
Decline pushups (elbows out)
Resisted shoulder press
Resisted upright pulls

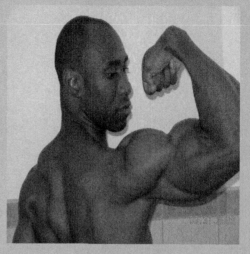

Day four repeat day one and continue the routine as follows till day six. Rest on day seven.

Week One: 3 sets each exercise, 15 reps bodyweight 15 reps resistance moves.

Week Two: 4 sets each exercise, 20 reps bodyweight 10-12 reps resistance moves.

Week Three: 3 sets each exercise, 30 reps bodyweight 7-9 reps resistance moves.

Week Four: 4 sets each exercise, 15-25 reps bodyweight 15 reps resistance moves. At the mid point at the end of your self resistance moves, perform a isometric (static) hold for 20-30 seconds using moderate tension.

CHAPTER 15

The Original Phase One
Workout
The Beginning
Phase Two

PHASE TWO
4 weeks

Day One

LEGS
One legged squats
Resisted leg extensions
Stiff-legged press
Resisted leg curls

CALVES
Slanted calve raises
Standing calve raises

UPPER CHEST
Decline pushups
Upper chess press

LOWER CHEST
Liederman press

TRICEPS
Resisted forward lateral press
Over head tricep press
Palm up tricep pressdown

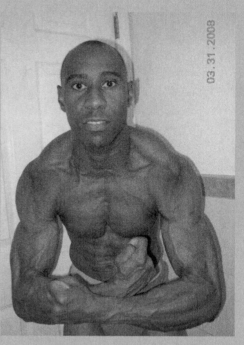

Marlon Messing Around.

Day Two

UPPER BACK
Across the body rows
Three chair dips
Resisted pulldowns
Stiff arm pulldown

UPPER TRAPS
Rear neck press
Side to side neck press

SHOULDERS
Decline pushups (elbows out)
Across the body lateral raises
Resisted forward raises
Across the body pulls

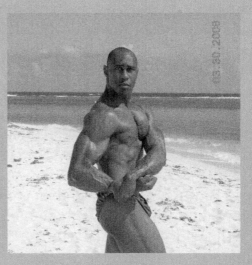

BICEPS
Palm up curl
Reverse curl
Resisted concentration curls

ABS
Reverse crunches
Across the body situps
Across the body side crunches

Day one and day two are alternated throughout the week for 6 days of training. 3 sets each exercise. 20 reps bodyweight moves, 10-12 reps resistance moves. Continue this phase for 4 weeks.

Acknowledgments

My greatest amount of gratitude goes out to my family for their support: Francis and Claris Birch (Grandparents), without them this book would have never been written. They are my greatest inspiration. My boy Kai Birch, that's my world.
My very good friend Elaine Mclean that have always stood at my side.
The appreciation you have given me throughout the years, I cannot repay. Marvin Wilson that has followed my boyhood dreams and never gave up on me. You are my brother. Camille Birch, Sharon Birch, and Neltrice Birch, The appreciation I have for all of you who assured me I can do it throughout the years. I Thank You. Also, I offer many thanks to everyone involved in the creation of this book from the very beginning to the very end: Dr. Desire Charles, Mr.Christie, Peter Goddard, Wanda Ebanks, Robert RPR, Maurice, Marcus, Steve Farr, all my followers and forum members. I can not thank you all enough. Infinite appreciation goes out to Mrs. Christie,Deborah Cervo, Damon and Tracey Paytner. Eduardo Tapia, Kris Morgan and Thiry Gordon. For their continuous support. Again, my never-ending love my Grandparents. For without their love, support, and positive outlook on life, they both made me what I am today. Thank you all for all the support throughout the years.

 Always in health and Strength

Marlon Birch